I Can Beat Obesity!

'Dr Nicola Davies has clearly understood that the key to losing weight is not only in the food we choose to eat, but also in our journey of self-discovery. This book is an excellent resource and self-help aid, and one I will find incredibly useful to use with my patients. I believe it will not only help them to understand the basic science behind obesity, but also enable them to have an insight into themselves and begin to understand the challenges they face to change their behaviour.'

– Jane DeVille-Almond, SRN SCM HV BA(Hons) PGcert, Independent Nurse Consultant and Chair of the British Obesity Society

'This is a great book which manages to combine the science of body weight and eating behaviour with extremely helpful tips on how to beat obesity, and is written in an accessible and inspiring way that should be a breath of fresh air to anyone who is struggling with their weight.'

– Jane Ogden, Professor in Health Psychology and author of several books on eating behaviour, including The Good Parenting Food Guide

'Dr Nicola Davies' latest book is an excellent read for both professionals and individuals alike. The approach is balanced between evidence and practical approaches for those wanting to understand the psychology of making a positive change to behaviours. The inclusion of self-reflection in each chapter enables the reader to maintain a connection and truly engage with the process of change.'

– Gil Barton, MSc PgCert FRSPH FHEA, health and well-being specialist and founder of The Healthy Workstyle Consultancy

'A refreshingly clear and well-written book providing insight into the origins and causes of obesity, before taking the reader through a structured and scientifically based set of strategies for losing weight. On the way, it provides a realistic guide to healthy weight. Highly recommended.'

– Dr Tony Cassidy, Professor of Child & Family Health Psychology at Ulster University

'A delightful book...your life will change.'

– Konstantia Keramidaki, health and wellness consultant

'Kudos to Dr Nicola Davies for having written an elucidative, intelligible and earnest guide for those who are considering embarking upon the journey to beat obesity. The book equips you to overcome this health hazard in an organised, hands-on fashion!'

– Dr Vandana Mathur (PhD Nutrition), nutrition and lifestyle consultant

'I've battled with weight for years, tried numerous diets, resorting to bariatric surgery. However, for continued success, I need to understand myself. This book is inspirational, very practical and encouraging and I believe it will be a great tool in helping people understand themselves and achieve the success they seek.'

– Patricia King, Accredited Counsellor/Supervisor
at Patricia King Counselling Services

'There is so much conflicting information out there – "Eat this, don't eat that" – Nicola's book instead focuses on the psychological barriers to change…a deeper understanding of self is key to long-term change.'

– Geraint Thomas, personal trainer and former professional rugby player

'Nicola Davies shows us the bigger picture of obesity… She is both a specialist and supporting companion, helping the reader prepare for change and encouraging self-reflection.'

– Mateusz Banaszkiewicz, health psychologist and Lecturer
at SWPS University of Social Sciences and Humanities

I Can Beat Obesity!

Finding the Motivation, Confidence and Skills to Lose Weight and Avoid Relapse

DR NICOLA DAVIES

Foreword by Jane DeVille-Almond

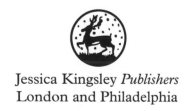

Jessica Kingsley *Publishers*
London and Philadelphia

The Readiness Ruler on page 51 is used with permission. Based on research conducted by The State Networks of Colorado Ambulatory Practices and Partners (SNOCAP-USA) under contract to the US Agency for Healthcare Research and Quality, Rockville, MD (Contract No. HHSA 290-2007-10008). The Stages of Change figure on page 57 is used with permission from www.smartrecovery.org. The Weight Efficacy Lifestyle questionnaire on page 67 is used with the permission of Gretchen Ames, PhD, ABPP. The Mood Diary on page 79 and Visual Mood Diary on page 80 are used with the permission of Carol Vivyan. The Eatwell Guide on page 117 is licensed under the Open Government Licence v3.0. Crown Copyright, Public Health England in association with the Welsh government, Food Standards Scotland and the Food Standards Agency in Northern Ireland.

First published in 2017
by Jessica Kingsley Publishers
73 Collier Street
London N1 9BE, UK
and
400 Market Street, Suite 400
Philadelphia, PA 19106, USA

www.jkp.com

Library of Congress Cataloging in Publication Data
A CIP catalog record for this book is available from the Library of Congress

British Library Cataloguing in Publication Data
A CIP catalogue record for this book is available from the British Library

ISBN 978 1 78592 153 7
eISBN 978 1 78450 420 5

Printed and bound in Great Britain

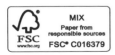

*This book is dedicated to my mother,
Pamela Davies, who struggled with obesity
for much of her life, and to others wishing to beat
obesity and weight-related problems. You can do it!*

Contents

Foreword

If you are reading this foreword, then it is probably not the first self-help obesity book you have ever picked up. In fact, there are currently over 32,000 books to be found on the Internet claiming to help you deal with your weight. Many of these offer a quick fix, radical diet or unrealistic change to your life. They claim to help you be slimmer, happier, healthier, better, more successful. You name it, there's a book out there professing to help you achieve it.

Despite training as a nurse in the 70s, it wasn't until my first serious involvement in obesity during the late 90s that I realised just how little I knew about the subject. I was convinced that all anyone wishing to lose weight should know is the simple rule of 'energy in, energy out'. If the energy in is greater than the energy out, then the likelihood is that you will get bigger and vice versa. This rule, of course, still stands the test of time, but I now realise that the real cause of obesity starts in our minds and with our attitudes towards ourselves.

Dr Nicola Davies has clearly understood that the key to losing weight is not only in the food we choose to eat, but also in our journey of self-discovery.

This book is an excellent resource and self-help aid, and one I will find incredibly useful to use with my patients. I believe it will not only help them begin to understand the basic science behind obesity, but also enable them to have an insight into themselves and begin to understand the challenges they face to change their behaviour.

Jane DeVille-Almond, SRN SCM HV BA(Hons) PGcert
Independent Nurse Consultant
Chair of the British Obesity Society

Acknowledgements

A huge Thank You to my biggest supporter, Alex Buckley, as well as to my publisher for believing in the value of this book. I would also like to extend my gratitude to Jane DeVille-Almond for her professional insights.

Disclaimer

Every effort has been made to ensure that the information contained in this book is correct, but it should not in any way be substituted for medical advice. I am a health psychologist and counsellor, but readers should always consult a qualified medical practitioner before making any major changes to their diet or physical activity. Neither the author nor the publisher takes responsibility for any consequences of any decision made as a result of the information contained in this book.

Preface

First of all, congratulations on picking up *I Can Beat Obesity!* because *you can beat it*, and by opening this book you are starting to believe in your ability to do just that. This is a huge step, so don't underestimate just how important this is for you and your future. By giving yourself permission to peek inside these pages, you have started to do one of the key actions that will help you beat obesity: you have started to look after yourself and to recognise that you deserve to be happy and healthy. Yes, happy and healthy. This isn't just about weight loss, but about being healthier — in mind and body. As you read this book, you will start to see that beating obesity isn't about going on a diet or starting a mad exercise routine. It's about being kind to yourself and learning to love and accept yourself. It is about working with, not against, your own mind and body.

In *I Can Beat Obesity!* we will take a journey of four parts:

- In Part One, we will arm you with the knowledge to beat obesity. I want you to understand the science behind obesity so that you are empowered to beat it if you choose to.

- In Part Two, we will prepare to beat obesity by exploring your readiness and confidence to take this journey.

- In Part Three, we will take action to beat obesity, exploring emotional, cognitive (thoughts), behavioural, social, dietary and physical well-being. These dimensions of your well-being are fundamental to beating obesity, because unless you feel worthy and able to achieve a healthier lifestyle, you are unlikely to achieve your goals. Have you ever wondered why so many people get trapped in yo-yo dieting? It's because they simply address their weight, rather than their whole self — and we are more than our weight. *You are more than your weight.*

- In Part Four, we will move beyond obesity and start to look at how you can accept yourself and start to focus on your future hopes and dreams.

Each chapter will start with information and finish by going 'Over to You!' In these 'Over to You!' sections, you will be able to complete some exercises to help cement your new knowledge and move you closer to your goal of beating obesity and, later, moving beyond obesity.

The approach in this workbook is based on the discipline of health psychology, which uses an understanding of human emotions and behaviours to help you achieve better health and well-being. I have a doctorate in Health Psychology and have experienced first-hand its power – personally and in my work – in assisting with the adoption of healthier behaviours and the cessation of unhealthy behaviours. I just wish I had studied the topic in such depth in time to help my mother, who struggled with obesity-related issues much of her adult life. Being close to my mother, I adopted many of her behaviours and also struggled with my weight as a child, but I was fortunate enough to be driven by a love of learning that led me to health psychology. I am now much healthier and much happier, and you can be too – just follow me and enjoy the journey towards a new you.

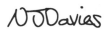

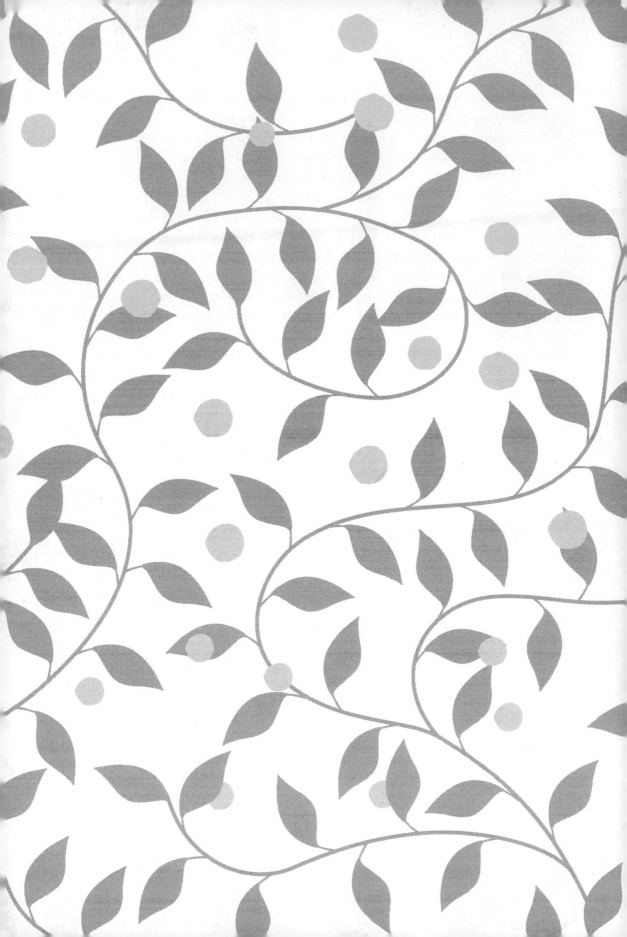

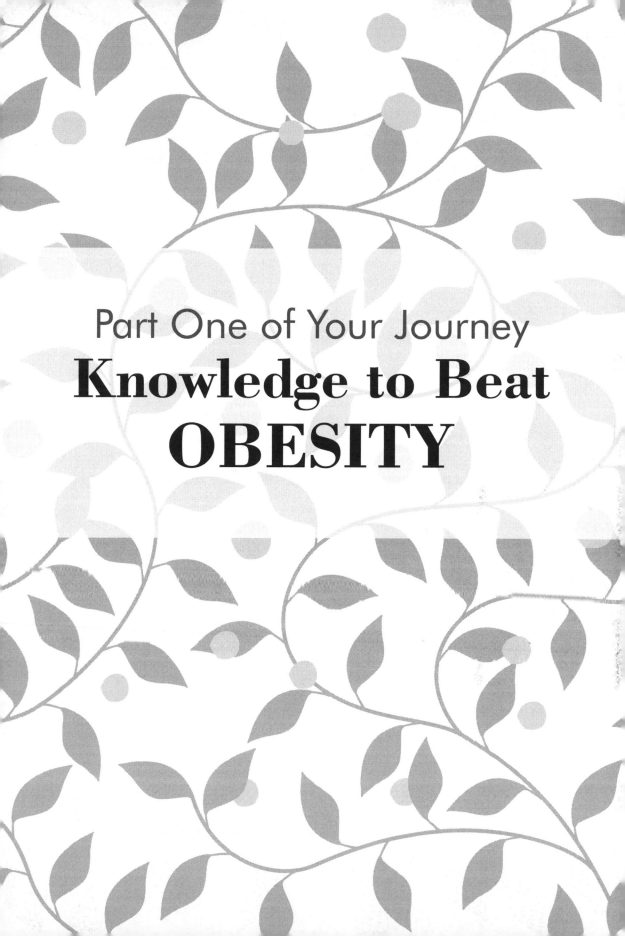

Part One of Your Journey

Knowledge to Beat OBESITY

Chapter 1

Understanding Obesity

> *Where ignorance is our master, there is no possibility of real peace.*
>
> Dalai Lama

Welcome to your journey to beating obesity! The first few chapters present a range of information, because in order to beat obesity you need to understand it. As a health psychologist, I am interested in the science of obesity and I want to share my knowledge with you to make you an expert on the subject. I believe that knowledge is power and I want you to have the power to make a healthier life for yourself. There is so much misinformation out there about weight and weight loss – possibly more than with any other topic. Sticking with these initial chapters will help replace some of this misinformation with evidence-based knowledge that you can use to pave your way forward.

The Obesity Taboo

Excess weight in the body has several, often undesirable, effects on a person's overall health and well-being. Despite this, it remains a taboo topic that is difficult for many to discuss. This is primarily due to the stigma of being obese. This book aims to help break the stigma of obesity by tackling it head-on – not skirting around the problem, but taking the bull by the horns to help you learn what obesity is, whether you have it and what you can do about it.

Jane DeVille-Almond, Chair of the British Obesity Society, once said, 'Having the confidence to raise the issue of weight with someone who is overweight or obese can be the first step to improving their health and reducing their risk of developing chronic health conditions in the future.'[1] However, it doesn't need another person to raise the issue of obesity with you. With a proper understanding of what the condition is all about, you can raise the issue with yourself to find out whether you are obese and what you can do to beat it.

What Is Obesity?

Put simply, obesity is the condition of having too much adipose tissue (also known as fat) stored in the body. The World Health Organization (WHO) defines obesity and overweight as 'abnormal or excessive fat accumulation that presents a risk to health'.[2] Its fundamental cause is an imbalance between energy consumed and energy expended.

With the global spotlight on obesity, 'obese' has become a term that is loosely used. So, first of all let's dispel some misconceptions about the condition.

✗ Overweight is the same as obesity.

Being overweight is not the same as being obese. Overweight may simply be due to having heavy bones or muscle mass, or even high body water content, but not necessarily fat. Obesity, on the other hand, refers only to having too much adipose tissue or fat in the body. Both conditions, however, refer to having weight or fat that is in excess of what is considered healthy for your height.

✗ An ideal weight is a healthy weight.

Some people assume that when their weight isn't their ideal weight, then they are unhealthy or 'too fat'. A healthy weight is computed based on your height, weight and other factors (which are discussed in the following subsection). On the other hand, your ideal weight is often based on your personal preference and how you want your physique to appear. For obese people, losing 5 or 10% of their weight can already be healthy (or healthier) because it can reduce the risk of developing certain health problems. So, always try to aim for a healthy weight, rather than your ideal weight – they aren't necessarily the same thing.

✘ **Obesity is detected through shrinking clothes and extra pounds.**

Some people assume they are overweight or obese when their clothes feel tighter and they need to shop for larger sizes, when the weighing scales show they've gained weight or when their waist feels wider than before. Although these signs show that you have gained some weight, they do not automatically mean you are obese.

How Common Is Obesity?

Obesity is extremely common, with data from 1975 to 2014 showing that it has risen dramatically over this 40-year period.[3] It has more than tripled in men and more than doubled in women. The problem is getting so serious that, globally, more people are obese than underweight and it is anticipated that one-fifth of the world will be obese by 2025.

In the UK in 2015, 24% of adults were obese and a further 36% overweight, making 60% of the adult population either obese or overweight.[4] In the US, the rate of obesity is even more alarming, with more than one-third of the US adult population being obese.[5]

Globally, obesity has more than doubled since 1980. In 2014, the WHO recorded 1.9 billion adults as being overweight, and 600 million of these were obese. These numbers are expected to keep on rising: it is estimated that, by 2050, 50% of the adult population will be obese.[6] The rate of obesity is escalating so fast that experts say being overweight will soon be the norm.

Am I Obese?

Do you think you are obese? Two of the most widely accepted tools for assessing obesity are body mass index (BMI) and waist circumference.

Body Mass Index (BMI)

BMI, which is the more commonly used tool to assess obesity, is a weight-for-height index.[7] Your weight in kilograms (kg) is divided by the square of your height in metres (kg/m^2). A BMI of 25 or more is considered overweight, and 30 or greater is considered obese.

Take some time to compute your own BMI – your weight in kilograms divided by the square of your height in metres – and compare your results with the table below to find out what your weight status is.

BMI	Weight status
Below 18.5	Underweight
18.5–24.9	Normal
25.0–29.9	Overweight
30.0–34.9	Obese (Class I – in a physically unhealthy condition and at a low to moderate risk of obesity-related health problems)
35.0–39.9	Morbidly obese (Class II – at high risk of obesity-related illnesses)
40.0 or greater	Extremely obese (Class III – at extremely high risk of obesity-related health problems that may lead to premature death)

Source: Adapted from the National Heart, Lung, and Blood Institute 2016[8]

Whatever your results, don't rely solely on this: BMI isn't necessarily accurate! Health experts are quick to use BMI as a tool to evaluate weight status, but many of them will also say that it isn't an accurate estimate.[9] Although it is calculated with the consideration that there are differences in people's heights, BMI cannot reflect weight due to body fat alone or the distribution of fat, and therefore it does not directly measure obesity. This explains why some athletes who are highly muscular are categorised as obese, even when they don't have excess body fat. Some critics argue that the BMI is an inaccurate description of the physiology of the person and is just a tool for insurance companies to charge higher premiums for people with higher BMIs.[10]

Waist Circumference

The second tool commonly used to measure obesity is waist circumference, which is simply a measurement of your waist. While weight circumference has traditionally been assessed based on gender, the new simple rule is that your waist circumference should be less than half of your height.[11]

Where do you fit in terms of weight circumference? To measure your own waist size, stand up straight and run a measuring tape around your middle area, just above the hipbones. Exhale and then measure your waist.

So, rather than relying on the more commonly used BMI, use the knowledge gained from both measures to help you assess whether you are obese or at risk of obesity. If you are still uncertain, it would be a good idea to seek expert input from your doctor or a dietician.

Know Your Fats

Now that you have a better idea of whether you are obese or not, let's take a look at the different types of body fat and those that you need to be most concerned about.

Body fat can be classified according to two locations – visceral or subcutaneous:

- **Visceral fat** is stored inside the belly area and wraps around the walls of internal organs, which means it can't easily be removed by typical diets or exercise. This type of fat increases the risk of developing serious health problems such as cardiovascular disease and diabetes.[12]

- **Subcutaneous fat** is found right beneath the skin and is what you can physically measure when taking your waist circumference – your 'love handles'. It isn't as dangerous as visceral fat, but when it comes to the belly area, both types of fat are present. A growing belly can be a sign that one or both types of fat are increasing in the stomach region, which is associated with an increased risk for stroke and various illnesses.[13]

Body fat, visceral or subcutaneous, is made up of fat cells, which fall under the domain of the endocrine system – the glands in your body that produce hormones and regulate your metabolism. Fat cells, together with other cells and tissues in the body, form your adipose tissue (also known as fat).[14] There are two kinds of adipose tissues – brown and white:

- **Brown adipose tissues (BAT)** are, as you might expect, dark brown in colour. They are linked with many blood vessels and are associated with calorie burning, heat production and energy balance. It's abundant among newborn babies, but diminishes as we age. It has also been found to be more abundant among people of normal weight, making it an attractive subject to study for scientists looking for weight management solutions.[15]

- **White adipose,** on the other hand, is responsible for storing energy and accumulates excessively in obesity. In a healthy body, muscles, adipose tissue and the liver absorb glucose (sugar) from the bloodstream. White adipose supports this process of glucose regulation, which in turn helps to reduce the risk of obesity and diabetes. However, when white adipose becomes excessively thick, its ability to help regulate glucose levels becomes disrupted.[16]

Over to You!

Now that you have a better understanding of obesity, reflect on the following question (being completely honest with yourself):

✎ **Am I obese? What have I learned from this chapter that has guided my answer to this question?**

_____

_____

_____

_____

_____

_____

_____

_____

If you have identified yourself as being obese and you want to change that, it can be useful to understand why you are obese. Move to Chapter 2 to explore this further.

Chapter 2

Why Am I Obese?

> Appetite is governed by our thoughts, but hunger is governed by the body.
>
> Clement Martin

Although BMI and waist circumference can be used to diagnose obesity, they don't reflect the multitude of factors involved in *why* you might be obese. Obesity can be understood better by looking at five factors: biological, behavioural, psychological, social and environmental.

1. Biological Factors

The biology of obesity involves the complex sensual and cognitive (your thoughts) responses that happen during food intake, which are triggered by the smell, texture, taste, temperature and appearance of food, and tell the brain to start or stop eating. Sometimes genetics and metabolism can also play a role.

Genetics

Genetic factors help to explain why people have different bodily responses when faced with the same food or when consuming the same amount of food. For example, people can have heritable sensitivities to hunger and external food cues.[1] The 'FTO gene' has also been linked to differing levels of energy expenditure and ability to control eating behaviour, both of which are associated with the development of obesity.[2] Although genetic factors can increase the likelihood of obesity, it is still low physical activity and high calorie intake that ultimately trigger genetic predispositions to obesity. Genetics can and does play a role in obesity, but healthy activity and eating practices help to control obesity for people of all genetic backgrounds and predispositions.

Metabolism

Metabolism is the chemical process by which we use and store food and water, so that we can grow, heal and make energy. Metabolism is largely controlled by the hormones that regulate appetite, the digestion and uptake of glucose, and the regulation and distribution of fat in the body.

Obesity may be caused by a hormonal imbalance – for example, hypothyroidism, a condition where the thyroid gland doesn't produce enough thyroid hormones. These thyroid hormones are responsible for regulating metabolism and use of energy, with some common symptoms associated with the condition being weight gain, high cholesterol, sleepiness, fatigue and muscle cramping. If you are sleepy and tired and your muscles cramp a lot, it is more difficult to be mobile and engage in physical activity. Also, when your body's metabolism is slow because of an underactive thyroid, it will be difficult to reduce the amount of food you eat and it will also be difficult for your body to use up the energy you take in. It is important to note, however, that although hypothyroidism can cause weight gain initially, once diagnosed and treated with thyroxine the thyroid becomes normal.

Another way in which metabolism and obesity are related is through the hormones that regulate appetite. Fat tissues and cells produce metabolism-regulating hormones, such as the appetite-suppressing hormone known as leptin. Interestingly, obese people have higher levels of leptin and yet their bodies don't seem to be sensitive to the hormone and therefore they don't feel full during and after meals.

Interestingly, as you lose weight, your metabolism will naturally slow down. This is because as your body size reduces, the less calories it needs to be maintained and therefore the less work your metabolism needs to do in order to pump energy around the body. In simple terms, there is less of you to maintain. This is why we need to keep our energy intake and output varied and adjust it as our weight fluctuates – in order to prevent a plateau when we still have more wait to lose or prevent further weight loss or gain when we have reached a weight we want to maintain.

2. Behavioural Factors

Our behaviours can have a huge influence on our weight.

Lifestyle

Lifestyle is the biggest behavioural factor when it comes to the rise in obesity. Just think of how much our lifestyle has changed over the years. Our ancestors used to exert huge amounts of energy foraging and hunting for their food – walking for miles, climbing hills, mountains and trees, all just to get food. If that doesn't sound tiring enough, they then had to carry all they had gathered back to their caves. This had to be done every single day because, unlike us, they couldn't store in bulk in their fridge or freezer. It would seem that obesity was unheard of then – most likely because people led active lifestyles and moderate-impact activities were part of their everyday routine.

When humans ceased to be nomadic and began to live in settled agricultural communities, they still maintained active lifestyles because they ploughed their fields and spent nearly all day every day engaged in physical activity such as herding their cattle, harvesting and planting. During the Industrial Revolution, when manufacturing became the foremost type of work, people still had a good amount of physical activity and walked most places.

Now, in the digital age, sitting down is something we all do regularly and much more than we need to. A sedentary lifestyle is just that – a lifestyle that involves a lot of sitting around. We sit when we eat our meals, we sit when watching television, we sit when we are on the computer, we sit in our cars or on the train or bus. While we are doing all this sitting, we aren't using the energy from the vast array of high-calorie food available to us, creating an imbalance of energy in versus energy out.

External Eating

External eating or impulse eating refers to eating that is triggered by external cues, and is often characterised by solo eating – eating by yourself – in the car, in the bath, while on the computer. External cues include time ('It's 12pm, so I must be ready for lunch'), seeing someone else eating, or passing a shop window displaying food. Certain activities or special occasions can also be associated with eating, such as snacking while watching television or viewing Christmas as a time for overindulgence.

In his book *Body Intelligence*, Edward Abramson proposes that the following behaviours could point to you being an external eater.[3] Tick those that apply to you.

✓ **I eat when I am around other people, even if I'm not hungry.**
　　□ Yes　　　□ No

✓ **If something smells good, I will try it.**
　　□ Yes　　　□ No

✓ **I will eat more of something that tastes good, even if I am full.**
　　□ Yes　　　□ No

✓ **I forget to eat when I lose track of time.**
　　□ Yes　　　□ No

✓ **I buy snacks or popcorn when I am at the cinema, even when I'm not hungry.**
　　□ Yes　　　□ No

✓ **I watch TV or read when I eat alone.**
　　□ Yes　　　□ No

✓ **I overeat on special occasions.**
　　□ Yes　　　□ No

We are all external eaters to a greater or lesser degree. Who hasn't overindulged just because it is Christmas or their birthday? External eating is only a problem if it is regular and involves many external cues.

3. Psychological Factors

According to the American Psychiatric Association (APA), our actions and inactions are often based on our thoughts and feelings.[4] In other words, the influence of emotions and psychological factors on eating must also be factored in when trying to understand obesity.

Attentional Bias

Attentional bias is when we pay greater attention to things that are more important or more pleasant for us. In the case of food, we might find it more pleasurable to look at a tasty cream cake than the plainer-looking lettuce leaf.

It is this attentional bias that often leads us to make dietary choices that are more in favour of desire than health. Equally, whereas the attention of one person strolling through the shops might be on fashion items or entertainment, images of confectionery, cakes and other sweet treats will leap out at a person on a diet and with an attentional bias for sweet foods.

Emotional or Comfort Eating

Emotional or comfort eating refers to the act of eating as a therapeutic tool. Emotional eaters turn to food to relieve stress and provide comfort. They treat their food as a reward instead of a means to satisfy their hunger. If you are an emotional eater, you may feel powerless to change the habit. You find yourself reaching for unhealthy desserts even when you are full. In a sense, you are trying to satisfy your emotional needs and not your biological needs.

Anyone can succumb to comfort eating, including those with otherwise healthy diets. This is especially the case when they are faced with stress that exceeds their tolerance level. Different people have different levels of stress tolerance – some may start to eat for comfort at the slightest hint of trouble, whereas others may endure a lot of emotional pressure before turning to food.

Although treating indulgent foods as a reward is not unhealthy in every instance, if you find yourself reaching for your favourite unhealthy snack with every small emotional trigger, you will soon find yourself using food as a primary coping tool. This is dangerous not just for your weight but also for your mind; it can be better in the long term to address your feelings of stress, sadness, loneliness, anger or boredom than to bury them in food. Burying emotions leads to a vicious cycle of emotion avoidance, which can be difficult to break.

To understand if you are an emotional eater, answer the following questions:

? Do you eat more when you feel stressed?
☐ Yes   ☐ No

? Do you eat when you are bored?
☐ Yes   ☐ No

? Do you eat when you aren't hungry?
☐ Yes   ☐ No

? Do you use food to reward yourself for personal achievements?
☐ Yes   ☐ No

? Do you feel safer when you eat?
☐ Yes   ☐ No

? Do you feel as if you have no control over your eating habits?
☐ Yes   ☐ No

Answering 'yes' to any of the above questions indicates you have a tendency towards emotional eating or eating for comfort. Note here that emotional eating can also be eating more when you are feeling positive – overeating can be your way of dealing with *any* heightened emotions, good or bad.

Binge Eating

Binge eating is a more extreme form of the symptoms that are created by emotional eating, and takes us into the realms of an eating disorder. It is defined as repeated episodes of eating excessive amounts of food (more than most other people) in a short period of time.[5] Like emotional eating, people who binge-eat often feel a lack of control when they are eating.

If you think you might have binge-eating disorder, it is likely that you also eat too quickly (even when you aren't hungry) and that you feel a huge amount of distress as a result of your eating-related behaviours and thoughts. People who binge-eat also feel great shame about their eating habits. This leads to secretive behaviour such as hiding food and keeping a personal stash of comfort foods, eating out of the view of others in cars and bathrooms, and embarking on periods of starvation dieting due to guilt.

To understand whether you might have binge-eating disorder, answer the following questions.

? Do you worry about the way you look when you are around other people?

☐ Yes ☐ No

? Does your appearance make you feel unhappy or ashamed?

☐ Yes ☐ No

? Do you worry about the amount of food that you eat?

☐ Yes ☐ No

? Do you often feel guilty or ashamed after eating?

☐ Yes ☐ No

? Do you find that you can't control your impulses when you are around food?

☐ Yes ☐ No

? Do you find yourself eating until you are very uncomfortable?

☐ Yes ☐ No

? If you break your diet with one food, do you give up and start eating other disallowed food?

☐ Yes ☐ No

? Do you embark on starvation plans when you don't eat anything for a period of time before binging again?

☐ Yes ☐ No

? **Do you often eat alone because you are ashamed of your eating habits?**

☐ Yes ☐ No

Answering these questions will help you to understand your relationship with food. All of these factors could be symptoms of binge-eating disorder. The more questions you answered 'yes' to, the greater the likelihood that you would be diagnosed with the condition. If you think there is some indication that you may be suffering from some or all of the symptoms of binge-eating disorder, you should consult a healthcare professional alongside doing your own self-help using this workbook. In Chapter 11, we will be exploring the role of professional support in your journey to beating obesity.

4. Social Factors

Social factors can also influence obesity in a number of ways.

Relationships

The link between social relationships and obesity has been the focus of some large studies. For instance, obesity tends to occur in social clusters.[6] Family members, colleagues and friends are part of the 'microenvironment' of a person, and these relationships often form the 'social facilitator of overeating'.[7] Indeed, it has been shown that food intake during meals eaten alone tends to be lower than during meals consumed in the presence of others. This behaviour can be due to the fact that when in the presence of others, physiological signals related to appetite, meal size and sense of fullness are overridden by social interactions. Also, the presence of other people at meal times lengthens the occasion, promoting greater food intake.[8]

Other studies have shown that when a sibling becomes obese, there is a 40% chance that another sibling will also become obese.[9] When a close friend becomes obese, the chance that another friend will also become obese rises to 57%. This can be explained by social network influences. When more people in your social network are obese, obesity is perceived as normal or acceptable, and weight gain is accepted as natural or inevitable. A counter-argument offered by some scientists is that the obesity cluster might be due to homophily – the tendency for people with the same body shape and size to become friends.[10]

5. Environmental Factors

Obesogenic Environments

The growing prevalence of obesity is clearly associated with both an increase in high-calorie, low-nutrient foods and a decline in physical activity. The physical and social environments in which we live play a role in shaping food choices and levels of physical activity. Where these environments play a role in promoting obesity, they are referred to as obesogenic environments.[11] For example, an obesogenic environment is one in which there is a real or perceived absence of safe and convenient opportunities to engage in physical activities such as walking or biking as alternatives to driving. In some places, purchasing healthier food options can be more difficult and expensive for poor and rural communities.

Light, Colour and Sound

Lighting significantly affects food consumption. It has been shown that dim lighting encourages a more relaxed attitude, where food is eaten with less self-consciousness.

Shops and cafés that display their desserts under those magnificent glass domes sell significantly more slices of cake than those who simply describe them on the menu, although menu writers do an exceptional job of engaging our senses with sensuously described dishes.

Noise also affects our eating behaviour. Relaxing music encourages us to linger, while a noisy environment encourages over-consumption as we often eat at a faster rate without realising how much we have eaten.

Colour and variety influence how much we eat too. Barbara Kahn, Professor of Marketing at the Wharton School, University of Pennsylvania, gave participants bowls of M&Ms filled with ten and seven colours respectively; the flavours for each colour were the same and there were 300 M&Ms in each bowl. After an hour, those who had the bowl with ten colours had eaten 27 more M&Ms than those with only seven colours.[12]

Over to You!

Now that you have a better understanding of various influences on obesity, reflect on the following questions (again, be completely honest with yourself):

✎ **If you are obese, why do you think you are that way? Write a brief summary, taking into consideration the various reasons discussed in this chapter.**

Biological factors _____

_____

_____

Behavioural factors _____

_____

_____

Psychological factors _____

_____

_____

Social factors _____

_____

_____

Environmental factors _____

_____

_____

✎ **Which of these factors are within my control?**

_____

_____

_____

_____

Do you want to take control of these factors and beat obesity? If you aren't certain, read Chapter 3 and then ask yourself this question again. If you know you want to beat it, Chapter 3 can help to cement your desire further, and the chapters that follow will provide the tools needed to make your desire a reality.

Chapter 3

Why Beat Obesity?

In 1991, researchers conducted a study involving adults who had lost 100 pounds or more after undergoing gastric restrictive surgery and were able to maintain their new weight for at least three years. The researchers investigated participants' perceptions about their previous morbidly obese condition, with alarming results. The participants viewed their previous state as having been distressing to the point that many of them would prefer to be normal weight with some major disability such as deafness, blindness, or even leg amputation, than return to their previous obese state. All participants also preferred to be normal weight rather than become a morbidly obese multi-millionaire.[1]

This isn't to scare you about being overweight or obese, but to let you know that obesity can lead to extremely distressing feelings, and that if you are experiencing them, you are not alone. Learning about how to beat obesity will first require an understanding of the importance of beating it.

Why Should I Be Concerned about Obesity?

Obesity can lead to several undesirable physical, social and psychological consequences, some of which you may already be feeling and others you might still not be aware of.

Physical Consequences

An obese person carries much more weight and stored energy than the body needs, which disrupts the regular and healthy metabolic flow in the body. Many obese people suffer from what is called 'metabolic syndrome', which is a complex set of risk factors including abdominal fat, increased blood cholesterol, insulin resistance, elevated blood pressure, elevation of blood components relating to inflammation, and elevated blood clotting factors.[2] These six risk factors, when grouped together, can dramatically raise your chances of developing diabetes or heart disease. However, any one of these risk factors alone is also a health concern that could lead to any or all of the following medical complications.

High Blood Pressure and Cardiovascular Disease

Obesity-related problems in the heart and blood vessels (cardiovascular system) can develop into cardiovascular diseases such as atherosclerosis (a build-up of plaque around the artery walls), coronary heart disease and heart failure.[3] These conditions are caused by increased blood pressure (hypertension) and accumulation of plaque on the walls of arteries that carry oxygen-rich blood from the heart to the rest of the body.

In overweight and obesity, much of the extra weight a person carries around is living adipose tissue (fat), which must be fed oxygen and nutrients by blood. This means the body needs more blood and the heart and blood vessels need to work much harder than in the body of a healthy-weight person. In addition, obesity causes the walls of arteries to become stiffer, making it harder for blood to be pushed through and therefore increasing blood pressure.[4]

Atherosclerosis can occur in any major artery in the body, and where it develops can vary from person to person. However, it is most common in the coronary arteries, which are the arteries that supply oxygenated blood to the muscles of the heart. This can result in coronary heart disease and, in severe cases, heart attack or heart failure.

Type 2 Diabetes

Type 2 diabetes is the most common type of diabetes, as well as one of the most serious health consequence associated with being overweight or obese. It was believed that Type 2 diabetes would only develop during adulthood, but it has been occurring in children more and more as obesity rates have increased.[5] In diabetes, the body experiences insulin resistance where it is unable to properly respond to, or make use of, the insulin that the body naturally produces. Insulin is necessary to maintain a healthy blood glucose level.

Insulin resistance is closely linked with obesity, having high levels of fat in the blood stream, and hypertension. The pancreas tries to produce more insulin to make up for the resistance, but often people with Type 2 diabetes need an external source of added insulin. Diabetes is highly likely to develop not only in morbidly obese people but also among moderately obese or overweight people.[6]

Cancer

Being overweight or obese is associated with an increased risk for developing various types of cancer, with excess weight being found to contribute to one in five cancer-related deaths.[7] Excess belly fat has been linked to cancers of the colon, rectum, uterus and pancreas. Excess body fat can contribute to the development of cancers of the oesophagus, kidney, gallbladder, liver, breast (for women after menopause) and prostate (for men).[8] Obese women are generally two or three times more likely to develop womb cancer than women of normal weight, and morbidly obese women are six times more likely.[9]

Complications During Pregnancy

In the UK, an estimated 15–20% of pregnant women are obese.[10] Maternal obesity, which is defined as when a pregnant woman's BMI is 30 or more during the first trimester, is a major concern. The risk of miscarriage during the first 12 weeks of pregnancy increases by 5%. Overweight and obese mothers are at risk of developing high blood pressure, blood clots, gestational diabetes and breastfeeding problems, while the baby is at risk of congenital anomalies, childhood obesity and respiratory problems.[11]

Joint Pain

Excess weight places more stress on the joints located in the knees and hips, causing joint pain that can worsen to become osteoarthritis. It has been found that the higher the BMI, the more severe the pain experienced in the joint. Pain in the knees causes a person to limp or fall frequently, which can also cause low back pain.

Respiratory Problems

Obesity can place extra weight on top of the chest area, which causes respiratory problems such as painful breathing, shortness of breath, excessive snoring and sleep apnoea (a sleep disorder where a person momentarily stops breathing while asleep, interrupting their normal sleeping pattern and causing drowsiness during the day).

Social Consequences

Weight Stigma and Discrimination

Unfortunately, in many Western cultures, there is pressure to look a certain way. Therefore, it is common for people with obesity to experience weight-related discrimination and stigma, which can negatively affect their mood and well-being.[12] Weight stigma and discrimination comes in varying degrees and from different people, including friends, family and strangers.

Reduced Lifestyle Options

Weight discrimination can also be expressed in terms of how some environments are designed in a way that places obese people at a disadvantage. When going shopping, for example, many shops will not sell larger sizes that fit obese people. When travelling on an airplane, obese people might need to purchase two seats in order to be comfortable.

Reduced Employment Opportunities

In the workplace, discrimination happens when overweight employees or applicants are denied a job or promotion, despite being qualified, because of their appearance. Research has shown that when application forms include a photo or video of the applicant, someone who is obese has a lower chance of being hired than a normal-weight counterpart.[13] Obese colleagues are also stereotyped as being less competent, sloppy and lacking in self-discipline and conscientiousness. They tend to be assigned to lower-paying jobs, and generally have less chance of enjoying better employment opportunities.

Healthcare Discrimination

Discriminatory attitudes have been documented among various healthcare professionals, all of who are prone to the same misconceptions as everyone else.[14] There are also instances where people who are obese aren't allowed certain treatments or where there is restriction on these treatments, such as hip replacement, knee surgery and other operations. It is important to note, however, that this isn't always discrimination but rather due to the heightened risk of anaesthetic complications in obese people. Also, some operations won't benefit those who are carrying excess weight.

Isolation

Stigma can eventually lead to obese people internalising the negative attitudes held against them, leading to self-hate and isolation.[15] Indeed, the negative attitudes of some people can lead those living with obesity to avoid social situations through fear of being judged. Therefore, they don't join social events where they could meet new people, and they may even avoid romantic relationships.

Psychological Consequences

Social factors such as weight stigma and discrimination increase the vulnerability of people who are obese to low self-esteem and self-worth, depression, anxiety and poor body image.[16] The psychological effects of obesity are detrimental in themselves, but often they become a greater cause for concern when they are paired with the physical and social consequences of obesity.

Body Dissatisfaction and Low Self-Esteem

With ideals of beauty being entangled with weight in many societies, including the UK, obese people, particularly young women, have a tendency to develop high body dissatisfaction and low self-esteem. They have a poorer perception of their health and capabilities, making them feel unable to participate in certain activities or to believe that they can live a fulfilling life.

Depression

Clinical depression is a psychological disorder in which a person's extreme feelings of sadness, anger, frustration or loss interfere with regular daily activities for a persistent period of time. Some of the symptoms include low or irritable mood, constantly feeling tired, difficulty sleeping, strong feelings of self-hate and worthlessness, and sometimes thoughts of suicide.

Depression has been found in people with obesity all over the world, even when there is no previous history of mental illness.[17] Depression and obesity tend to feed off each other in a detrimental way, with one prompting and perpetuating the other. One study found that obese people had a 55% increased risk of developing depression and depressed people had a 58% increased risk of developing obesity.[18]

Anxiety

Anxiety is another common psychological disorder associated with obesity, and studies have found that the likelihood of developing anxiety disorders increases as BMI increases.[19]

Anxiety disorders are characterised by having an intense and excessive feeling of worry, fear or terror that can interfere with daily activities. The feeling of anxiety is difficult to control and is often disproportionate to the actual level of danger or concern, and it can quickly escalate into a panic attack.[20] As a result, people suffering with an anxiety disorder avoid the things or places that trigger their panic.

Extreme anxiety can lead to the development of specific mood disorders such as panic disorder and agoraphobia (the extreme fear of crowded places). Many obese people suffer from a specific type of anxiety called social anxiety, whereby they avoid entering social situations for fear that their weight will become a subject of ridicule, such as being unable to fit into an airplane seat or damaging a restaurant chair. Social anxiety drives people to isolate themselves.

Low Quality of Life

Obesity can lead people to believe that they are unfit to take part in or enjoy the activities life has to offer. Furthermore, in many cases the condition itself stands in the way of the person's functional mobility – their capability to move around in the environment and participate in daily activities. With the extra weight, as well as the physical and psychological complications linked with being obese, some obese people can't enjoy the simplest activities such as going for a stroll or even playing with children or grandchildren. Chronic pain caused by some of the obesity-related physical illnesses can be enough to restrict the movement and enjoyment of obese people. This often results in reduced quality of life because they cannot fully engage in activities they enjoy.[21]

Over to You!

In this chapter, you have gained a broader understanding of the negative effects of obesity and the need to minimise the related risks to your health, relationships, career and quality of life. Now that you know why you might want to beat the condition, take some time to reflect on the following questions:

✎ **Do I sometimes experience weight discrimination and have weight-related negative feelings? When and where does discrimination usually happen and how does it make me feel?**

_____

_____

_____

_____

_____

✎ **What physical ailments or pains do I experience that are related to my weight? How do they affect my life?**

_____

_____

_____

_____

_____

✎ Do I want to beat obesity and what are my personal reasons for wanting to beat it?

_____

_____

_____

_____

_____

✎ Own your desire to beat obesity by completing the following sentence and reading it whenever you start to waver in your resolve:

I want to beat obesity because _____

_____

_____

_____

_____

_____

_____

✎ Using the scale below, how much on a scale of 0 to 10 do I want to beat obesity? (0 represents a very low desire and 10 a very high desire.)

```
├──┼──┼──┼──┼──┼──┼──┼──┼──┼──┤
0   1   2   3   4   5   6   7   8   9   10
```

If you weren't sure at the beginning of this chapter if you wanted to beat obesity, it is likely that you now have a number of reasons to motivate yourself. The next question is: *How?* Read Chapter 4 and take the first steps towards turning your desire for good health, opportunities and a fruitful life into a reality.

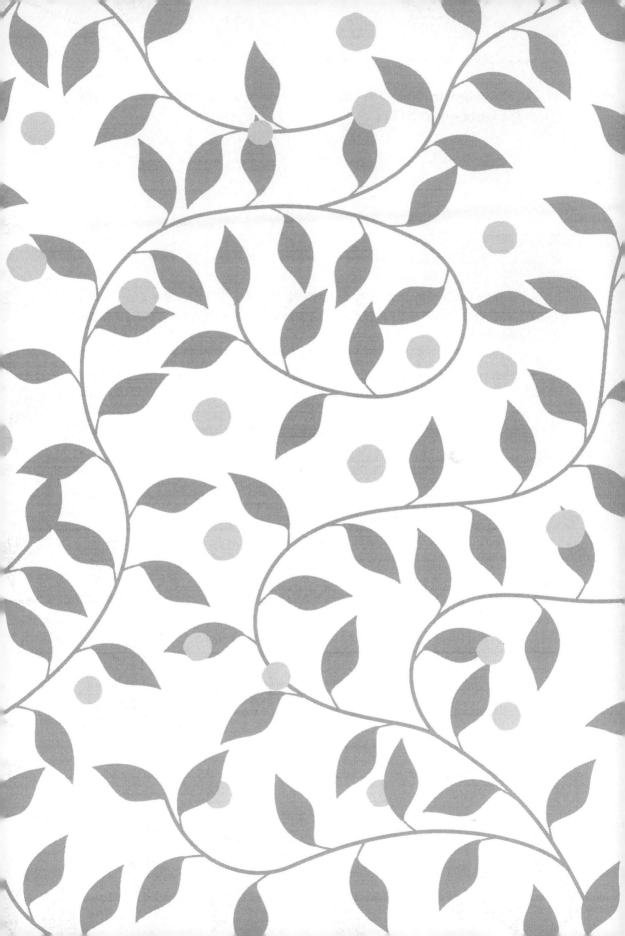

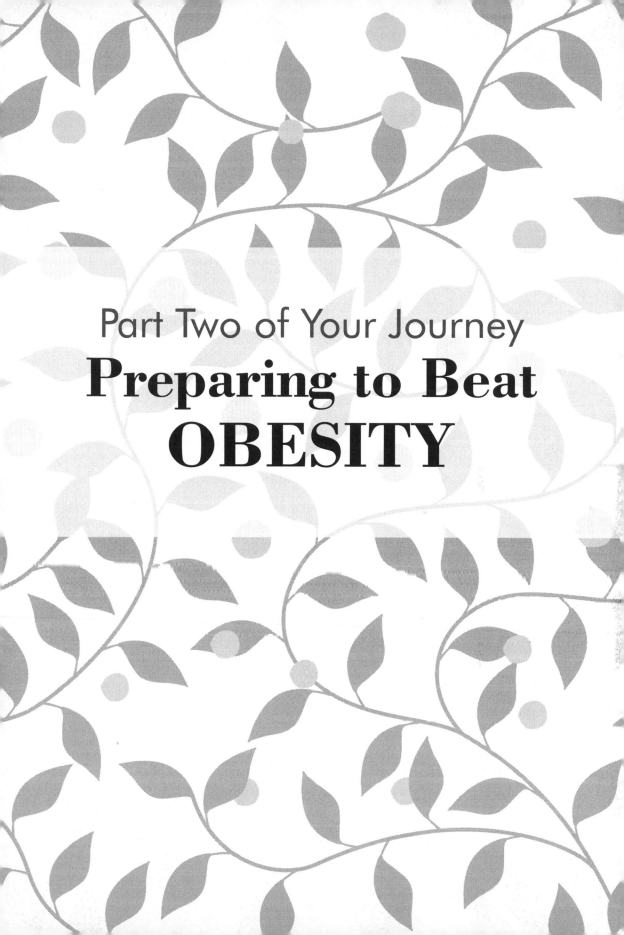

Part Two of Your Journey
Preparing to Beat
OBESITY

Chapter 4

Beating Obesity

> The first step toward success is taken when you refuse to be a captive of the environment in which you first find yourself.
>
> Mark Caine

When we speak of beating obesity, it's common for people to assume that we are simply referring to losing weight. For cases of morbid obesity where the life of a person is already at risk, doctors might prescribe bariatric surgery, which could take the form of a gastric bypass or a gastric band. However, you don't have to wait until surgery becomes the medically prescribed option for you to lose weight; you can take control yourself – now. Furthermore, in this chapter you will learn that losing weight is only part of the solution to beating obesity. This is about *you*, your *health*, your *happiness* and your overall *well-being*.

Diet, Exercise or Both?

The two most common solutions to losing weight are dieting and increasing physical activity. Dieting refers to limiting the amount or kind of calories you consume for a certain period of time. Physical activity increases your metabolic rate, builds muscle, burns fat and increases flexibility and stamina.

Exercising can sound like a lot of work, but there is some reassuring news. A 2014 study compared the effectiveness of diet only, exercise only and the combination of diet and exercise in weight loss. It was found that in the short term the amount of weight lost was similar for the diet-only plan and the combined diet-and-exercise plan. However, in the long term, weight loss was more effective under the combined plan as opposed to the diet-only or exercise-only plan.[1] In other words, there is no need to worry about physical activity for the time being, especially if this is putting you off taking steps to beat obesity; dieting rather than strenuous exercise is more crucial at the start of your journey to beat obesity.

This isn't to dismiss the importance of physical activity; it has many other benefits besides weight management. However, if it is fear of physical activity that is preventing you from taking on the challenge to beat obesity, remember that you can start to integrate exercise into your lifestyle when you are ready. The chances are that as you gain a healthier diet and start to build your self-esteem, you will naturally start wanting to do more physically because you will have more energy. So, yes, physical activity is important, but at the beginning of your journey it isn't the be-all and end-all – it is something to aim for.

Dieting isn't the be-all and end-all either, however. As you probably already know, changing to a healthier eating plan is one thing and sticking to it is a whole other matter. Many people abandon their diet programme halfway through or, for those who do commit to it, are still at risk of gaining back all the weight. Diet, along with exercise, may be enough for you to lose weight, but it may not be enough to beat obesity in the long term.

What Does it Take to Beat Obesity?

So, what is beating obesity really about? Beating obesity goes far beyond losing weight. It requires embracing a lifestyle change – one that begins with the mind. It isn't just about changing what you eat or what you do, but about *wanting* to make changes to how you live the rest of your life. To jump-start your journey towards beating obesity, you need to begin by looking closely at your attitudes and behaviours. From there, you need to develop the *willingness*, *readiness* and *confidence* to make the changes required to beat obesity.

Be Willing

Change can't happen if you aren't open to accepting that there may be certain areas in your life that need changing. Do you really want to live a healthier life? If the answer is yes, then you need to be *willing* to look at various aspects of your life, such as the habits and routines that are contributing towards an unhealthy lifestyle. Next, you need to be *willing* to take steps towards reducing or getting rid of these destructive habits.

Start with your mind and cut down what is called 'mental fat'. This is made up of the unhealthy attitudes and habits that get in the way of sustained weight loss.[2] Some examples of mental fat include the following:

1. **Giving in to deeply ingrained unhealthy eating rituals:** 'I know I should eat this high-fibre vegetable, but this fried chicken looks delicious. Maybe I can take one piece of the chicken and a little of the vegetables. Just this once.'

2. **Fearing what others might say about your attempts at making a serious change:** 'I've always been the chubby person everyone likes to hug. If I lose weight, who will I be?' or 'If I start this, I don't want other people seeing me try in case I fail.'

3. **Postponing lifestyle change plans and blaming it on work demands, peer pressure or family issues:** 'I want to seriously sit down and plan my diet and exercise, but I have so many deadlines at work and I need my sugar fix to get all the work done on time.'

If you don't feel ready to examine and identify your unhealthy mental patterns and attitudes, you may find it difficult to motivate yourself to accept and maintain change. In which case, any changes you make will only yield short-term results.

Be Ready

After identifying the attitudes and behaviours around food, work, friends and self that are creating an unhealthy cycle, you can begin to reflect on small changes that can be introduced in place of those bad habits. You can then ask yourself: *Do I understand how much of my time and mental strength it will take to see these changes through?* To answer this, you need to be equipped with the right information. The more you learn and become familiar with what it means to be healthy, the better you will be at choosing which options are best for you. This is one of the aims of this book – to empower you with the information needed to make the decisions that are best for you.

Ultimately, being ready means having a plan or, at the very least, having the possible answers at hand. To plan, you need to be prepared to welcome new information about health that could change the way you look at food, physical activity, relationships and how you treat yourself.

Be Confident

Readiness and willingness can get one foot in the door and be catalysts for developing a healthy lifestyle. Sticking to a plan and getting the other foot moving, however, requires *confidence*. How certain are you that you can move from thinking about change towards applying what you've learned and actually *making* the change?

Beating obesity requires that you are confident in your ability to handle the physical, psychological and social demands of change. You must be able to start, succeed at and sustain a healthier lifestyle within the context of the kind of job you have, the people you spend time with and the responsibilities you need to fulfil.

Part of being confident is being realistic and working within your strengths and limitations. For instance, some frameworks for dieting and exercise encourage people to detach from their regular life. If you were to follow the well-known cabbage soup diet, for example, you would need to withdraw from doing anything that requires energy and you would probably start underperforming at work and home.

Remember to be patient and realistic so that, although you are focused on your plan to beat obesity, you are also prepared to experience potential setbacks. Don't think of them as failures. Failure doesn't exist, not if you take a lesson from your setback and use it to help you move forward.

Losing weight is important, but in the context of living a healthy life it is only a by-product. The goal is not so much to lose weight but to have the kind of mindset that makes you *ready*, *willing* and *confident* to introduce small but meaningful changes into your daily routine, making it easier for you to choose health every time.

Beating obesity is about building your emotional, social, dietary and physical well-being – a challenge to make an overall lifestyle change that doesn't prevent you from performing your roles at home, at work and in your personal life. Instead, it allows you to perform them better.

Over to You!

This chapter has explained how beating obesity goes beyond diet and exercise. It is also about a deep mental shift that requires you to be *ready*, *willing* and *confident* to make a genuine change to your overall lifestyle and, ultimately, to be kind to yourself. Reflect on the following questions.

✎ What makes up my 'mental fat'? How do these habits, attitudes and behaviours contribute towards an unhealthy lifestyle?

_____

_____

_____

_____

_____

✎ How ready am I to beat obesity? (Use the readiness ruler below to measure your level of readiness on a scale of 0 to 10, with 10 being the readiest.)

My level of readiness:

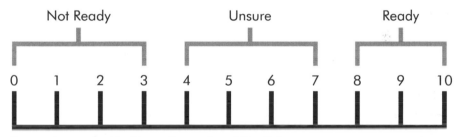

Source: Agency for Healthcare Research and Quality[3]

✎ Am I willing to commit to the necessary changes to beat obesity? (Use the willingness scale below to measure your level of willingness on a scale of 0 to 10, with 10 being the most willing.)

My level of willingness:

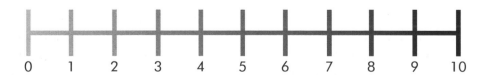

✎ Am I motivated to commit to the necessary changes to beat obesity? (Use the motivation scale below to measure your level of motivation on a scale of 0 to 10, with 10 being the most motivated.)

My level of motivation:

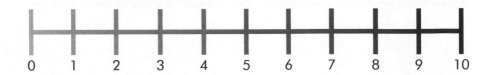

0   1   2   3   4   5   6   7   8   9   10

✎ Do I believe that I can beat obesity? Do I understand what it takes psychologically, behaviourally, physically and socially?

_____

_____

_____

_____

_____

_____

Beating obesity requires a shift in the way you treat your body. Lacking the willingness to change may indicate that you've already given up before even getting started. However, you have the power to decide against that and to motivate yourself to kick-start a change in your lifestyle. Chapter 5 will help you to determine how ready you are to beat obesity and how to orient yourself towards the healthy-living mindset.

Chapter 5

Are You Ready?

> Determine that the thing can and shall be done,
> and then we shall find the way.
>
> Abraham Lincoln

Health psychologists use something known as the Readiness to Change scale to help people change unhealthy behaviours, including behaviours related to obesity. Understanding and using this tool yourself can help you to progress through your journey to beat obesity. In particular, if you have been unsuccessful in changing your lifestyle in the past, this tool can help you to evaluate the environmental and psychological obstacles that may be in your way. Remember what we discussed about failure not existing if you learn from it. This comes into play here: by using the Readiness to Change scale you can turn failure into success.

What Is the Readiness to Change Scale?

The Readiness to Change scale involves several stages, and answering a few questions can help you understand which stage you are in when it comes to changing your lifestyle for the better.[1]

There are six main stages in the Readiness to Change scale, as shown in the figure on the next page. Which one do you think you are in?

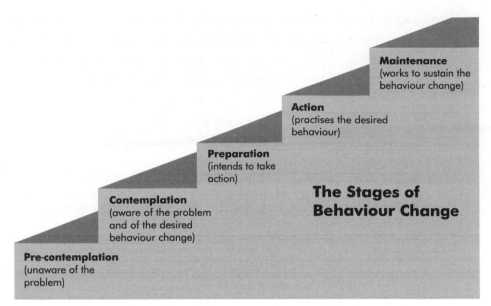

Source: Prochaska and DiClemente[2]

Stage 1: Pre-Contemplation

People who are in the pre-contemplation stage are not yet ready to take action. They aren't able to recognise the problem (in this case, obesity), even though everyone around them can. Those stuck in the pre-contemplation stage resist change, and small setbacks demoralise them enough to give up on any preparation for change. To move past this stage, you need to accept that demoralisation is natural at this point of the change process and that the situation is not hopeless; change is possible. Remember, you just need to be *ready*, *willing* and *confident*.

Stage 2: Contemplation

By recognising the problem and seeking solutions, you have moved into the contemplation stage. In this case, the problem is obesity and the solution is to change your lifestyle. If you are in this stage, you want to start on the road to change and have realised that, with active effort, you can start to move towards your goal of beating obesity. However, at this stage you are still struggling; you want to change your lifestyle, but you can't clearly see the specific obstacles in your way in order to reach your end goal.

There is a real risk of stagnating in this stage and many people do so if they don't make the effort to understand the obstacles to lifestyle change that are specific to them. At this stage, you may be making vague plans for change, but not taking any action. To move past this stage, it is important to understand the specifics of why you are obese. Think back to Chapter 2 where you explored the factors involved in your obesity. To help you gain further insight and to move beyond the contemplation stage, try to answer the following questions:

- How is being obese affecting my life?

- What makes it hard to manage my weight?

- How do I think my life will improve if I reach my health goals?

- What could I do if I reach my health goals that I am not able to do now?

Stage 3: Preparation

At this stage, you are planning to make changes imminently (within a month). Preparation is very important to the success of your goals and there are several steps that can be taken at this point to increase your chances of moving steadily through the stages of change.

First, it is important to make your goals public. Tell your friends and family about your intentions – but only those whom you trust to be supportive. Making your goals public within your support network will allow you to draw on their help and guidance when you are under stress. Including trusted family and friends in your plans can also help to lessen any hesitancy you may be feeling and will help to motivate you to move forward.

The preparation stage is also when you put your decisions for change down in stone and set yourself some clear and achievable goals; we will explore this in more detail in Chapter 7.

You can take your time with the preparation stage, but set a firm date for when you will move on to the next stage. Whenever you choose to move forward, preparation is key. People who don't plan properly often find they are unable to overcome any challenges they face in the next stage of change – action.

Stage 4: Action

Once you have a plan and a time frame, you can move into the action stage of lifestyle change. This is when you start to make your goals real. You need to enter this stage with a clear picture of what is required on a day-to-day basis and how you are going to deal with small challenges. Remember that there will be setbacks on the way, and it is important to have a plan for how to deal with them effectively, so that they don't trip you up completely.

This stage will require commitment in both energy and time. The action stage is when you will start to notice improvements. Keep track of your achievements, and throughout this stage ask yourself the following questions in order to reinforce the positive effects of your efforts:

- What changes have I noticed in my body?

- How have changes in my weight affected the way I feel about myself?

- Am I able to do more now?

- How do I picture myself six months from now if I continue this journey?

- How will family and friends react when I reach my goal?

Stage 5: Maintenance

Although action may feel like the hardest and most important part of the Readiness to Change stages, maintenance is just as important. If maintenance isn't carried out properly, you will risk moving back to the first stage of change. In order to maintain the new, healthier you, try to reinforce the factors that led to you moving successfully through the action stage. Spend time focusing on the positive effects of your new lifestyle – the way you look and feel, but, more importantly, the health and psychological benefits. Think about the positive impact of your new lifestyle on those around you, such as your family and friends. Reflecting in this way will help you stick to new healthy habits.

Moving forward, you have navigated the maintenance stage successfully if you can answer 'yes' to this question:

? **Have I maintained my lifestyle change for at least six months?**

☐ Yes ☐ No

By this stage, you will have built up healthy habits that will help you to keep yourself strong in the face of temptation. It is now up to you whether you relapse to old behaviours or enter what is known as the 'graduation' or 'termination' stage (see figure below).[3]

The Stages of Change

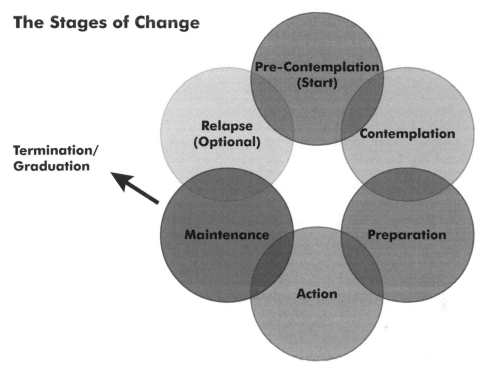

Source: SMART Recovery[4]

Stage 6: Termination/Graduation

In the termination stage, a person is no longer tempted to revert to previous, unhealthy behaviours, and therefore further action and change is no longer needed. In effect, the person has full confidence in maintaining the behaviour needed to sustain a healthy or desired weight. Even in the face of temptation or adversity, a person in this stage does not revert to unhealthy habits in order to cope.

For those making efforts to beat obesity, the termination stage is often more of an ideal or goal than an actual state of being. When it comes to something as natural and necessary as eating, practising healthy behaviour typically requires continued vigilance or maintenance. Sustaining healthy eating and activity habits may require a lifetime of maintenance. This is particularly true with the increase in obesogenic environments.

The goal is to move through these stages steadily to avoid stagnating in any particular stage. By understanding the Readiness to Change stages and which stage you are in, you will be able to organise and enact your new lifestyle effectively. Ultimately, it's important to stay positive and keep your desired goals in sight so that you can move forward through each stage with excitement and resolve.

Over to You!

✎ Answer the following three questions to gain a better idea of where you fall on the Readiness to Change scale:

- **Have I tried to lose weight in the last month?**
    ☐ Yes ☐ No

- **Have I tried to avoid gaining weight in the last month?**
    ☐ Yes ☐ No

- **Am I prepared to actively try to lose weight and reach my goal in six months?**
    ☐ Yes ☐ No

If you answered 'no' to all of the preceding questions, you are stuck in the pre-contemplation stage. The very fact that you are reading this book, however, is a good indicator that you are ready for change and are, at the very least, in the contemplation stage. If you answered 'yes' to the first two questions, congratulations – you are at the preparation stage. Indeed, the very fact that you have made it to the 'Preparing to Beat Obesity' section of this workbook suggests you are in this stage.

✎ So, how can I now move from preparation to action? What do I need to do to help myself take that next step? If you aren't sure, think about a time in the past when you had a difficult task ahead of you and what you did to support yourself in progressing forwards.

_____

_____

_____

_____

_____

_____

_____

_____

Once you have your answer, move on to the next question.

✎ Knowing *what* you need to do is all well and good, but even better is also knowing *when* you are going to act on your plans. So, when and how am I going to implement the above in order to move towards the action stage?

_____

_____

_____

_____

_____

_____

When you are ready to beat obesity, move on to Chapter 6 to take a closer look at your confidence to beat obesity.

Chapter 6

Are You Confident?

> *Believe you can and you're halfway there.*
>
> Theodore Roosevelt

Your state of mind is incredibly important when it comes to successfully adopting and maintaining behavioural changes that will improve your health and well-being. So, now that you have a better idea of how *ready* you are to beat obesity, let's take a look at how *confident* you are – your self-efficacy.

What is Self-Efficacy?

Your self-efficacy is your belief in yourself and your ability to achieve your goals – in this case, your healthy lifestyle and beating obesity goals. Understanding the role of self-efficacy in the uptake of healthy behaviours has been useful in the treatment and self-management of eating disorders, smoking, alcohol consumption, pain and chronic diseases.

The concept of self-efficacy is best known through the work of the psychologist Albert Bandura.[1] For Bandura, self-efficacy is the extent to which a person believes they are capable of performing certain activities well enough to influence other events and processes that affect their lives. Perceptions of self-efficacy shape how people feel, think, motivate themselves and behave. In terms of tackling obesity, self-efficacy refers to your confidence in your ability to adopt and sustain the positive changes in behaviour needed to maintain a healthier lifestyle, especially in the face of challenges that might tempt you to revert to unhealthy behaviours.

Self-efficacy is not just blind confidence in your abilities, but a conscious, reasoned appraisal of your capacity to act based on previous experiences. Self-efficacy is also not the same as self-esteem, which is a much more general concept. Self-efficacy refers to beliefs in *specific* abilities to complete *specific* tasks, rather than to general feelings of self-worth, although the two may certainly be related.

People with high self-efficacy will typically believe they can achieve a difficult task to a high level of competency. People with a low sense of self-efficacy with respect to a difficult task will typically focus on potential obstacles, personal deficiencies and all kinds of adverse outcomes, rather than concentrate on how to best accomplish the task. They also engage in more negative self-talk, which reinforces their low self-efficacy. People with low self-efficacy are at greater risk of depression, which can make beating obesity even more difficult.

The Benefits of Self-Efficacy

Since self-efficacy is rooted in how we perceive ourselves, it can be measured quite easily via questionnaires. The most commonly used questionnaire for people trying to beat obesity is the Weight Efficacy Lifestyle (WEL) questionnaire, which rates your confidence to exhibit a specific behaviour in various 'high-risk' situations.[2]

Let's use the questionnaire to take a quick look at your own level of self-efficacy. Use this readiness ruler below to rate your confidence about the questions presented in the table on the next page.

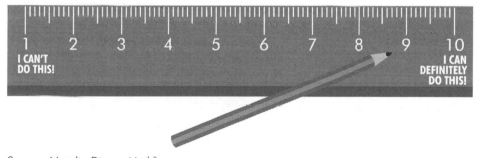

Source: Natalie Digate Muth[3]

Self-efficacy question	Confidence number (1 to 10)
I can resist overeating when I am anxious.	
I can resist overeating at the weekend.	
I can resist overeating when I am tired.	
I can resist overeating when I am watching TV.	
I can resist overeating when I am depressed.	
I can resist overeating when I am in a social setting.	
I can resist overeating when I am angry.	
I can resist overeating when others are pressuring me to eat.	

Source: Natalie Digate Muth[4]

Using such questionnaires, researchers have shown significant links between self-efficacy and declining BMI within obesity treatment programmes that include a psychological and behavioural component.[5]

Here is some more evidence of just how powerful self-efficacy can be when it comes to beating obesity:

- In an 18-month study, increases in self-efficacy over time improved weight loss.[6]

- In a six-month trial among early post-menopausal women who received a balanced meal plan with reduced calorie intake, individuals with higher self-efficacy were able to lose more weight.[7] The results are particularly significant because early post-menopausal women are at high risk of gaining weight and have greater difficulty losing weight than women who are either younger or older.

Research also indicates that previous experience of being unsuccessful at beating obesity is important in shaping a person's self-efficacy for tackling obesity again. However, one study showed that an increase in confidence was more important in lowering weight than starting out with high confidence.[8]

This suggests that even people with low initial self-efficacy can build up their confidence in a way that will empower them to beat obesity. So, if you have low self-efficacy when it comes to beating obesity, don't worry – you can build it up; in fact, the exercises in this workbook are designed to help you do just that.

How Can I Improve My Self-Efficacy?

Perceptions of self-efficacy are developed, or learned, through experience over time. In particular, there are four factors that shape self-efficacy and can be used to improve success at beating obesity: mastery experiences, vicarious experiences, verbal persuasion and physiological states.

Mastery Experiences

Mastery experiences are experiences of success at adopting some form of behaviour that is seen as difficult to accomplish. These experiences of past success are thought to be the most important factor in creating high self-efficacy.[9] Success builds confidence in a person's ability to effect change in their life; not succeeding undermines that confidence, until sufficient mastery has been experienced to allow a person to overcome setbacks. In some cases, it may not be lack of success that hinders development of self-efficacy, but previous negative experiences; for example, a previous injury sustained during physical activity may lead to fear of injury or re-injury if physical activity is recommended for beating obesity.

Achieving mastery of a particular behaviour, such as not comfort eating, is no small feat and should be approached through setting realistic, attainable goals; goals that are too ambitious can lead to a sense of failure and diminished self-efficacy. Goals can be reassessed periodically, as you get comfortable with individual successes, to ensure self-efficacy is not based solely on an absence of 'failure' but on success over adversity.

Vicarious Experiences

Vicarious experiences are those felt through the observation of another person's actions. Observing other people achieve success in tackling obesity can allow us to see our capacity for similar forms of success. For vicarious experience to be helpful in addressing personal struggles, the person whose behaviour is being modelled must not only be seen as having achieved success after attempting something difficult, but they must also have similar characteristics such as age, class, gender, personal history and present challenges; the greater the similarity, the greater the impact their success will have on you.[10] Without the similarity of circumstances, it is not realistic to think: 'If they can do it, then so can I.'

You do need to be careful when you are observing the behaviour of others, however; don't set yourself up for the unachievable. Ideally, the person whose behaviour you are modelling will be a peer or social equal. Furthermore, the goal of modelling needs to be improvement of self rather than trying to be like someone else. The important lesson is learning determination and perseverance against obstacles.

Verbal Persuasion

Verbal persuasion refers to positive encouragement that boosts a sense of capacity to initiate and sustain change, especially when encountering obstacles. When verbal persuasion succeeds in enabling a person to meet their lifestyle goals through hard times, this builds mastery experiences. However, it is not helpful when praise is unwarranted or exaggerated; it has to be genuine and realistic. In addition, it is easier to undermine self-efficacy through criticism than to build self-efficacy through encouragement. So not being self-critical is just as important as giving yourself praise.

When seeking sources of verbal persuasion, it is important to find people with similar experiences to yourself, such as others who have struggled with obesity and/or the changing of lifestyle. Professional counsellors are also an important source of verbal persuasion as they have experience in guiding people through difficult times by providing mental strategies to deal with any mixed feelings you might have regarding change. They can also help you to find alternatives to negative self-talk. Sometimes, it just takes a trusted person who has faith in your abilities to persevere and succeed, even if they haven't experienced similar lifestyle-related problems.

Physiological States

Physiological states such as tiredness, anxiety and pain have a profound effect on our mood and emotions, which in turn affect our confidence. Confidence can also change depending on the particular stressors you are facing at a particular time. You may have faith in your ability to accomplish something until the situation changes, and it may be as simple as someone negative from your past walking into the room.

So how do these four components of building self-efficacy all fit together? Programmes designed to help people beat obesity, such as Weight Watchers and Slimming World, demonstrate how the interaction of these four components can help with weight loss and maintenance. A key aspect of successful programmes is the *mastery experience* of achieving positive results and the *vicarious experience* and *verbal persuasion* of being with similar others who provide encouragement and feedback. Such programmes also incorporate skills development for dealing with barriers to beating obesity, including how to deal with various *physiological states* that might hinder your progress.

Working on raising your self-efficacy is only one part of a solution to obesity, but it is one of the most important parts. It puts your sense of control in the foreground, challenging you to seek solutions and maintain successes. Seeing improvement in how you think and behave, and especially in your capacity to direct your own change, is a more meaningful indicator of success than simply measuring weight loss by the pound.

Over to You!

✎ I believe I can beat obesity because:

In the past, I've done something more difficult than losing weight, such as _____

_____

_____

_____

_____

I have role models to look up to who have also beaten obesity, such as _____

_____

_____

_____

_____

✎ I can be kind to myself and encourage myself to meet my goals by telling myself (only tick those you can tell yourself with sincerity):

☐ I can do this; I know I can.

☐ I'll take it one meal at a time, one day at a time.

☐ I can beat obesity to regain my _____

☐ I can beat obesity so that I can feel _____ about myself.

☐ I can beat obesity so that I can keep up with my _____

As you build up your confidence, you will start to feel able to set some clear goals to work towards, as discussed in Chapter 7.

Chapter 7

What Are Your Goals?

> Setting goals is the first step in turning the invisible into the visible.
>
> Tony Robbins

The importance of setting goals as part of your journey to beat obesity has been mentioned throughout this book. The goals you choose for beating obesity will need to address what actions you want to take to effect personal change (e.g. changing diet and activity levels), and what outcomes you want to achieve (e.g. lowered weight and improved health).

Setting goals for beating obesity can be understood in six simple steps:[1]

- Step 1: **Recognising** a need for change in particular behaviours that have contributed to your obesity.

- Step 2: **Establishing** appropriate, personally tailored goals based on a realistic understanding of your capacities.

- Step 3: **Implementing** the behaviours needed to achieve your goals.

- Step 4: **Monitoring** your progress by keeping notes of your strengths and weaknesses as you endeavour to beat obesity.

- Step 5: **Rewarding** yourself for achieving goals.

- Step 6: **Assessing** the need to revise your goals, or add new goals, in light of the information you gain from monitoring your journey.

You need to be ready and motivated to embark on these steps. Motivation to achieve goals is especially important for long-term maintenance of healthier behaviour. If you have made it to this chapter, then it is likely that you are ready and motivated.

The Benefits of Goal Setting

There has been a significant increase over the last two decades in research on the role of setting goals in the promotion of better health. There is now clinical evidence that goal setting can improve the uptake of healthier eating and greater physical activity in order to reduce the risk of obesity and obesity-related chronic diseases. One study even concluded that because goal setting was shown to promote dietary change, training for goal setting should be added to nutrition-based interventions.[2]

In a review of 13 studies assessing the effectiveness of goal-setting interventions for promoting positive dietary and activity behaviour against a group in which there was no goal setting, eight studies showed that goal setting can facilitate positive changes in dietary and activity behaviour.[3]

More specifically, setting goals has been shown to motivate higher achievement by encouraging us to try harder, with greater concentration on the task at hand, and for a longer period. This increased effort, concentration, and persistence is most consistently achieved when goals are highly specific, difficult to achieve, and set for a short time frame, requiring effort immediately rather than allowing for postponement.

Setting Your Goals

When setting goals, make sure they are **S**pecific, **M**easurable, **A**chievable, **R**ealistic and **T**ime-bound – they need to be SMART.[4]

Be Specific and Measurable

Specifying the exact details of the tasks needed to complete a goal ensures you know the necessary steps to reaching your goal. Specific goals reduce resistance to change, so they are more likely to be achieved; vague goals are easier to avoid and more likely to result in returning to the habits you have been trying so hard to change.[5]

To be specific, goals ideally need to address one action and one object, or one activity being planned for and monitored. For example, if you wish to take a 15-minute walk three times a week and stretch for five minutes afterwards, it is easier to track this as two separate goals since they are separate challenges. Just by completing one of them, you will build up your sense of accomplishment and confidence to achieve the next goal. You will have proven to yourself that you can set a goal and stick to it.

For goals focused on altering complex behaviour patterns associated with obesity, it can be difficult to know which details to focus on because there are many specific behaviours, contexts, time frames and other factors that need to be accounted for. Therefore, having a goal of being more physically active may be precise, but it doesn't provide any guidance on *how* to achieve that goal. Think carefully and honestly about the range of behaviours you are willing and able to change in order to be more active. For example, are you willing to have a ten-minute stroll every morning after breakfast, or is it more feasible to commit to a longer walk once a week?

Also, in order for a goal to be specific, it must be measurable. For example, if you want to increase physical activity, you must set a goal that can be measured in time (minutes), or in distance (kilometres) or number of repetitions or days of the week.

Make Goals Achievable

Setting goals that are realistic is not about *lowering* your expectations, but increasing the likelihood of the mastery experiences we discussed in Chapter 6 – these are important to boosting your confidence and keeping you on track. Setting realistic goals also helps with the maintenance of healthy behaviours over the long term. Realistic goals for beating obesity should be achievable, but difficult enough to require a real challenge and effect real change.

Be Realistic and Time-Bound

When setting your 'beating obesity goals', it is better to aim for a healthier lifestyle than one-time weight loss. Realistic goals for tackling obesity are largely focused on behaviours that you have the ability to change through personal effort, concentration and persistence. For example, it is better to seek to eat more fruit than to eliminate a specific food group.

In addition, it is important to set both long-term and short-term goals, where the short-term goals will help you to meet your long-term goals. Achieving a healthier lifestyle is a long-term goal, but the short-term goals to help you along the way might be adding two more minutes a week to your afternoon walks, having an apple a day, reading up on nutrition and so on. Achieving these small goals will give you a sense of accomplishment because you are moving towards the desired, larger goal.

Having a well-thought-out set of long-term and short-term goals makes it easier to keep track of and focus on the specific behaviours needed to achieve a healthier lifestyle. Well-specified short-term goals are particularly important since they provide more immediate feedback (remember the power of verbal persuasion and praise discussed in Chapter 6).

In line with setting realistic goals, the goals you set need to be based on your levels of commitment, confidence and knowledge, as well as your own personal circumstances such as available time and resources. Since personal circumstances can change, it can be helpful to stage the introduction of new goals for times that are most appropriate and add room for exceptions.

For example, experts recommend that kicking bad habits is far easier with a change in environment or setting.[6] So, if you are used to overeating in a specific room, make sure you start eating your food in another room – a room that has become part of the new you – at least at the outset of your journey to beat obesity. You need to ensure that any triggers that might get in the way of your goals are identified in advance, so that you can put a strategy in place to overcome them.

Assessing the Need to Revise Goals

Assessing achievement of goals and the need to revise goals or add new ones is essential in ensuring the goal-setting process is effective in beating obesity over the long term. Assessment is not just about checking to see if goals are met, but careful consideration of how you can better meet your goals and what goals are best suited to your circumstances, based on your experience to date with achieving goals. Have experiences with goal setting led to greater satisfaction and quality of life? Or perhaps your experiences have led to low self-esteem? If the former, then you can dissect that past experience to see what you did right and to incorporate it into your new goals. If the latter, maybe you now have a better understanding of whether you were perhaps setting unrealistic goals that resulted in making you feel bad because you couldn't achieve them.

Assessment of goal achievement can come from your own review of your experiences, although it is often helpful to seek feedback from another person whom you trust. Both assessment of goal achievements and provision of rewards for successful achievement have been identified as vital to fostering greater motivation and confidence, ultimately leading to healthier choices of behaviour.

Over to You!

Now that you know more about the different aspects of goal setting that can help you beat obesity, take some time to consider your own goals.

✎ **My long-term goal is:**

_____

_____

_____

_____

_____

_____

✎ **The short-term goals that will help me towards my long-term goal are:**

_____

_____

_____

_____

_____

_____

✎ **My plan of action for achieving these goals is:**

_____

_____

_____

_____

_____

_____

_____

_____

_____

_____

_____

_____

✎ I am going to start working towards these goals on _____
(add specific dates to start working towards each of your short-term goals):

Short-term goal	The date I will start

Are you feeling more prepared to beat obesity – more ready, willing and confident, with clear goals to achieve? If so, follow me to the next part of your journey.

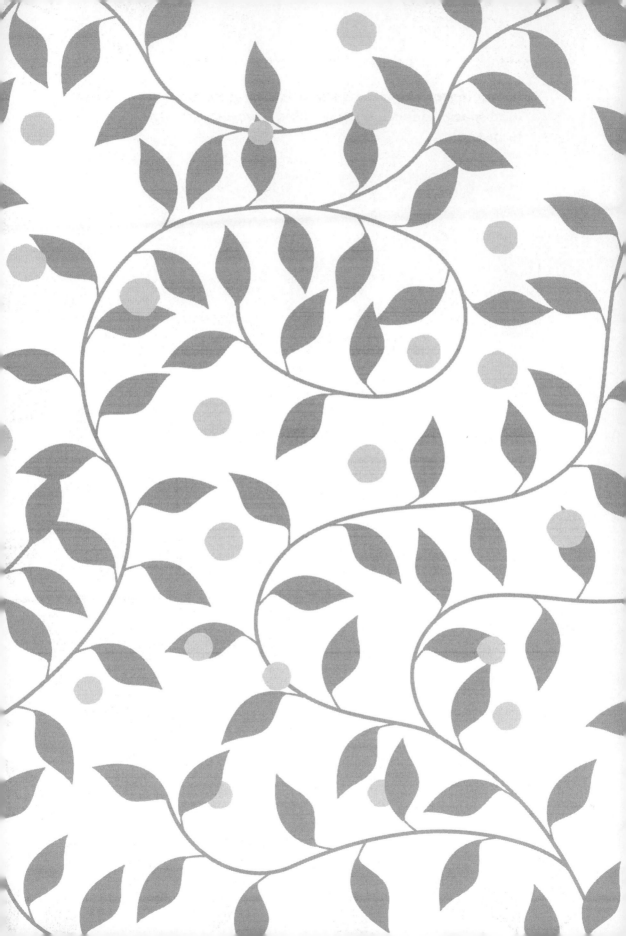

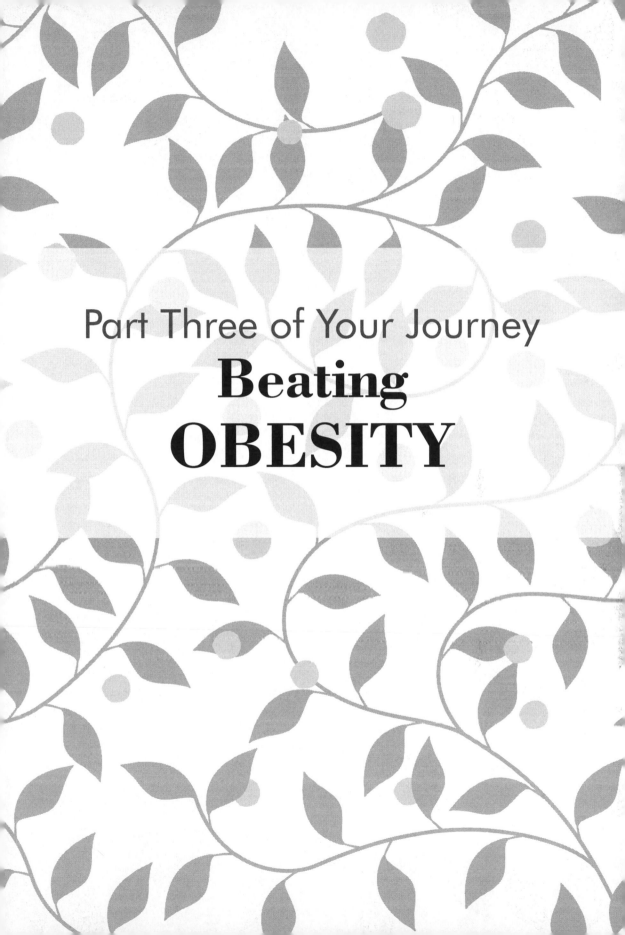

Part Three of Your Journey
Beating
OBESITY

Chapter 8

Your Emotional Well-Being

> " *Although the world is full of suffering, it is also full of the overcoming of it.*
>
> Helen Keller "

Beating obesity isn't just about looking after your body; it's also about taking care of your mind. Indeed, weight and emotional health can be so entangled that it is difficult to tackle one without the other. Let's take a closer look at the link between obesity and emotional well-being, as well as your own emotions and how you can work with them in ways that will help you beat obesity.

Emotions and Eating

How does overeating or eating unhealthy foods relate to emotions? Most often, it is because we use food to compensate for something, to deal with major life changes or to cope with stress, fear, boredom, sadness or anger; food can make us feel better in such circumstances.[1] This is, in part, because eating certain foods such as sweets, cheeses, chocolates and some meats produces the 'feel-good' chemical dopamine. To get that positive feeling again and again, people develop the repetitive practice of eating the same kind of food, which eventually disrupts the body's normal pathways for feeling hunger and fullness. Constantly seeking dopamine-releasing foods will eventually lead to overeating and weight gain.[2] Foods that are especially high in sugar can even create an addictive cycle.

According to the American Psychological Association (APA), many adults frequently overeat because of stress.[3] If an overweight person is confronted with a problem or finds themselves in a stressful situation, eating comfort foods can serve as a distraction. However, the APA also reports that almost half of adults who overeat or eat unhealthy foods to cope with emotions feel disappointed in themselves and their bodies afterwards.[4] In other words, the benefits of reaching for dopamine-enhancing foods in the face of adversity are short term and can actually exacerbate your emotional distress in the long term.

The Emotional Journey of Achieving a Healthy Lifestyle

If you don't keep your emotions in check, they can get the better of you. This is especially true if you attempt to make lifestyle changes when you are emotionally vulnerable. How you feel can either boost or get in the way of your healthy lifestyle plans. Your negative emotions can eat away at your motivation to beat obesity, and depressive symptoms such as low mood, hopelessness and helplessness, when coupled with high personal expectations and a low tolerance for stress, can sidetrack you from your goals to achieve health and well-being.

Negative emotions can also fuel a negative body image, making your initial steps of achieving a healthier lifestyle feel like a struggle. You may have very high expectations for yourself, and once you observe that you aren't reaching your desired goals as quickly as you would like, you may become frustrated, angry and insecure. This is why it is so important to learn how to moderate your emotions, so that your health efforts aren't derailed. Let's take a look at some tools that can help you with this.

Keeping Your Emotions in Check

Beating obesity can be an emotional roller-coaster, and having negative moods will be unavoidable at times. In order to deal with your feelings in a way that will prevent relapse into unhealthy behaviours, you need to find a way to express your emotions. It's important to be honest with yourself and to recognise and process feelings no matter how negative they may be. To facilitate this, there are steps you can take to deal with your emotions and to regain control.[5] For example, you could make use of a mood diary, reflective journal, relaxation techniques or mindfulness practice.

Mood Diary

A mood diary is a tool to chart your emotions over a period of time. It can be as simple as noting down your most prominent emotions per day over a month, or it can be as detailed as charting your moods, anxiety levels, changes in routine, eating, energy levels and sleeping patterns each day.

What is important is that this tool is used to record your feelings as you beat obesity, to potentially reveal emotional patterns, mood and behaviour fluctuations, and specific sources of stress. A mood diary can help you detect and manage mood swings and maintain positive emotional habits such as self-restraint. When you are aware of your emotions, you can be in a more stable position to make decisions, reducing the likelihood of falling into old and unhealthy habits. Having a record of your moods can also help guide consultations with a health expert if you choose to get one on board.

Mood diaries are available as free online tools, such as the MedHelp Mood Tracker[6] or Mood Panda,[7] but you can also make your own by following these steps:

1. Decide on the items you will be recording (general mood, anxiety, depression, irritability, stress, etc.). You can choose as many as you can realistically observe and monitor.

2. Choose how often you will be recording each item (per day, twice a day, every other day, on every occasion that you feel an emotion strongly).

3. Create a rating system apt for each item. For example, you can rate anxiety from 1 to 5, where 1 is extremely low anxiety and 5 is extremely high.

4. You could include a comments area where you can write down phrases, thoughts or feelings you had for the day or while experiencing a particular emotion.

5. Sum up your ratings per item per week or month depending on your preference and try to identify patterns in your moods and behaviours. If you stay on track with your lifestyle goals, your mood diary should reveal the progress of your emotional health over time.

Below is an example of a simple mood diary to help you chart your moods, emotions, thoughts and feelings.

Mood Diary

Day and time	Mood/emotion Rate intensity of emotion 0–100%	Comments Example: What was happening, where, who with? What went through your mind (thoughts, images)? What were you doing just before and/or after you felt this way?

Source: Carol Vivyan[8]

If you are more visual, the mood diary below might be more appealing:

Visual Mood Diary

Monday	☹ ☺ ☺	+ Good things today:
	1 2 3 4 5 6 7 8 9 10	− Bad things today:
Tuesday	☹ ☺ ☺	+ Good things today:
	1 2 3 4 5 6 7 8 9 10	− Bad things today:
Wednesday	☹ ☺ ☺	+ Good things today:
	1 2 3 4 5 6 7 8 9 10	− Bad things today:
Thursday	☹ ☺ ☺	+ Good things today:
	1 2 3 4 5 6 7 8 9 10	− Bad things today:
Friday	☹ ☺ ☺	+ Good things today:
	1 2 3 4 5 6 7 8 9 10	− Bad things today:
Saturday	☹ ☺ ☺	+ Good things today:
	1 2 3 4 5 6 7 8 9 10	− Bad things today:
Sunday	☹ ☺ ☺	+ Good things today:
	1 2 3 4 5 6 7 8 9 10	− Bad things today:

Source: Carol Vivyan[9]

Journalling

A mood diary is a ledger of your moods over a period of time to reveal patterns. A journal, on the other hand, can be more useful if you want to go deeper into understanding the quality and nature of your emotions. Journalling is a reflective practice; not only do you list your emotions, but you also identify which events triggered the emotions, as well as how and why the events had such an impact on you. You can also evaluate your reaction to various situations and determine how you might better deal with similar situations in the future. You can clarify your thoughts and emotions and begin to see things from a different perspective, which often helps with problem solving and decision making. You also get to know yourself on a deeper level.[10]

Journalling isn't only a way to release emotions; it is also a scientifically proven tool to help you process the strong emotions related to your goal of beating obesity. Studies suggest that people with weight problems who journal about aspects relating to their weight loss goals lose twice as much weight as those who don't keep a journal.[11]

To start journalling, decide on what platform you will use. Some people prefer using a notebook and pen while others consider blogging. The choice is up to you; what would benefit you the most – privacy or sharing? If you choose the blogging option, it is a good idea to have your own private journal too, so that you have somewhere you don't feel the need to hold back.

Once you have a journal set up, ask yourself some questions to jump-start your reflective thinking:

- How do I feel about life?

- How do I see my future?

- If I could talk to my younger self, what would I say?

- What are my regrets?

- What are my hopes and dreams?

- What do I hope to get out of journalling?

Your journal is for everything and anything you want to explore, so make the most of it.

Relaxation Techniques

Negative feelings and stress can prompt you to overeat or eat unhealthy, sugary junk foods. Relaxation techniques, on the other hand, can help diffuse stress levels and curb cravings, ultimately empowering you to cope better in stressful situations. In one study exploring the impact of relaxation training on emotional eating, 60 obese women who suffered from emotional eating took part in a three-week relaxation intervention.[12] Relaxation reduced anxiety levels, depressive symptoms and emotional eating habits, and improved confidence among the women, which further facilitated their long-term weight management.

Examples of relaxation techniques include:

- meditation

- deep breathing

- massage

- yoga

- tai chi

- listening to music.

Can you think of any others to add to the list?

Not only do relaxation techniques have many health benefits, but they also promote a feeling of overall well-being and help you keep a positive outlook. There are different techniques and schools of yoga, deep breathing, mindfulness and relaxation. All of them can help you focus, remain calm and become more aware of your body. Consistent engagement with these health practices will enable you to have a better understanding of your body's needs and help you gain greater self-acceptance.

Mindfulness Practice

Mindfulness is a special kind of meditative practice in which you learn to pay active and close attention to your body, breathing, thoughts, environment and experiences in a non-judgemental manner.[13] Whether the experience is negative or positive is irrelevant; mindfulness is about recognising the experience and being fully present, and not about rejecting or holding on to the experience.

In recent years, mindfulness has caught the attention of many health experts. Among obesity specialists, mindfulness-based interventions are believed to be effective in controlling emotional eating, binge eating and external eating.[14] If practised correctly, mindfulness can cultivate emotional balance, self-acceptance and a better relationship with yourself and your body.

In a 2008 case study, a mindfulness-based intervention was introduced to someone who was morbidly obese and wanted a lifestyle change.[15] Interestingly, the results showed that the individual was able to cut his weight down from 315 pounds to 171 pounds. He was able to increase his physical activity, eat healthier foods and practise self-control whenever the urge to overeat came up. He was also able to maintain his wellness at one-year follow-up.

Mindfulness can last as long as 60 minutes or be as brief as three minutes. For beginners, 10–15 minutes should be enough. There are also variations to this practice, but there are three basic aspects you can focus on: body, breath and thoughts. Here's a mindfulness exercise for you to try.

1. First, relate to the body by sitting on a comfortable chair with your feet firmly on the ground.

2. Place your hands on your lap and relax your shoulders. Keep your back straight but not stiff.

3. You can keep your eyes open or closed.

4. Start to focus your awareness on the sensations, the aches, the curves and crevices of the body.

5. Next, place more attention on your breathing. Don't change the manner of your breathing. Simply inhale and exhale as naturally as possible and feel the breath come in and out.

6. Visualise the breath entering your nose, travelling around the body and leaving your body.

7. Lastly, bring your awareness to your thoughts, which could be memories, fantasies, plans for the following day or something you saw while scanning through social media. There is no need to get rid of these kinds of thoughts; rather, be an observer of your thoughts. However, make sure to bring your attention back if you drift off and forget that you are in the middle of a mindful experience. Importantly, don't be frustrated by interrupting thoughts – merely let them float through your mind on a cloud; accept that they are present and let them pass.

Another useful mindfulness tool for when you are feeling emotionally overwhelmed is presented in the box on the next page.

Feeling overwhelmed? Try this mindfulness exercise – stop, focus, release

Every time you find yourself dwelling on the past or worrying about the future, remember these three words:

- **Stop.** Stop what you're doing. Stop thinking about things you have no control over at the moment. Stop trying to do everything at once. Stop taking on more than you can handle. Stop rushing, stressing and planning. Stop allowing yourself to get distracted. Just stop.

- **Focus.** Focus on the present. Focus on doing one thing at a time and do it well. Focus on what people are saying to you and not what you want to say or should have said. Focus on every task as if it is the most important thing you can do in that particular moment.

- **Release.** Release any thoughts that have nothing to do with the present moment. Release your tension. If there are tasks you need to do that you don't have time for because you are focusing on the present, just let them go. Make sure you get the most urgent and important tasks done first and release the rest.

Keep repeating these three words to yourself as often as you need to: stop, focus, release.

Over to You!

This chapter explained how much power your emotions can have on your health. If you choose to monitor and take charge of your feelings, you can work with your emotions to help you beat obesity. Furthermore, by using the right tools – such as a mood diary, journal, relaxation techniques and mindfulness practice – you can develop greater awareness about your emotions and your body. Take a moment to reflect honestly on the following questions:

✎ How do stress, frustration, sadness, anger and insecurity affect your eating habits, self-esteem and motivation?

_____

_____

_____

_____

_____

✎ Make one entry for a journal about your thoughts and feelings right now, in this moment.

_____

_____

_____

_____

_____

_____

_____

_____

_____

_____

_____

_____

_____

_____

_____

✎ Perform 15 minutes of mindful meditation (set an alarm so that you don't have to worry about time). What feelings were you able to process? How did it make you more aware of your body and emotions?

_____

_____

_____

_____

_____

_____

_____

_____

_____

_____

_____

_____

_____

_____

You now have some tools to help safeguard your emotional well-being, but positive feelings cannot be sustained without a focused and positive-thinking mind. Chapter 9 will look at the role of your cognitive well-being – your thoughts – on the success of your journey towards beating obesity.

Chapter 9

Your Cognitive (Thoughts) Well-Being

> " *The only person you are destined to become is the person you decide to be.*
>
> Ralph Waldo Emerson "

When it comes to our thoughts, the mind can create a powerful internal environment that is either helpful or crippling. As with emotions, thoughts can also play a huge role in both the onset and maintenance of obesity – and, of course, in beating obesity.[1] The good news is that the mind can be influenced and you can train it to work with you rather than against you.

Cognitive Distortions

Unhealthy thinking patterns, also known as cognitive distortions or biases, can give rise to incorrect assumptions about who you are (e.g. 'I have always been the big one in the family') and what you can do (e.g. 'I don't have the willpower to stop comfort eating'). Such thoughts can be deeply embedded mental habits that must be broken. They act as fuel for depression, anxiety and feelings of low self-worth.

There are a variety of cognitive distortions that might be making it more difficult for you to beat obesity.[2] Take a look at the following descriptions to see if you can relate to any of them. For those you can relate to, there are some tips for breaking free from these self-destructive ways of thinking.

Black and White Thinking

Thinking in terms of diet and food being categorically good/bad or healthy/ unhealthy, or otherwise looking at them in extremes, is called black and white thinking.[3] Although it can help you shorten the list of foods you can readily eat, fast-track your dietary decision making and help you practise restraint in your food intake, this mentality is a strict and unforgiving all-or-nothing approach. It sets you up for feelings of failure and shame.

Anyone trying to beat obesity will sometimes go off track. This is understandable, expected, and normal. However, if black and white thinkers violate their lifestyle plan even once, they consider the incident to be a complete and utter failure in their efforts to beat obesity. A single episode of 'falling off the wagon' is taken as an indication that they have completely returned to old, unhealthy habits and will never be able to get back on track. As a result, they abandon their goals and return to their old lifestyle.[4]

Black and white thinking is polarised thinking where the only two options are you are healthy or you are unhealthy, which is not a reflection of reality. Thinking in extremes exposes you to having unrealistic expectations. For example, you may think enjoying a piece of birthday cake or taking a physical rest are signs of weakness, and so you push yourself to keep on going even if you are tired, burned out or utterly disinterested. Instead of feeling confident that you are in control of your health and your life, you might feel as if you are being deprived and punished.

How to Fix Black and White Thinking

Success is gradual. Begin by adopting a flexible frame of mind. Exercising a flexible type of restraint allows you to eat foods that have a higher-than-normal (compared with your dietary goals) fat or sugar content, but only once in a while to satisfy your cravings. This can be a more successful approach than depriving yourself entirely of all the foods you enjoy. More flexible rules are more realistic, and are a reflection of how much you trust yourself. Consider a single episode of binge eating as a lapse in your routine and as an opportunity to learn, rather than a relapse into your old lifestyle.

As Tarek Hamid explains in his book *Thinking in Circles about Obesity: Applying Systems Thinking to Weight Management*, thinking in black and white terms makes decision making easier, but a person's reality is broad – with plenty of room for middle ground.[5]

Black and white thinking can also appear in how strongly you fixate on a number on the weighing scale, thinking that if you don't achieve a specific number, then you are at the 'bad' and 'unhealthy' end of the spectrum. Thinking this way can limit your perspective, lead you to feeling constantly dismayed and result in you discrediting any achievements you have made so far.

To develop a flexible mindset, celebrate both your small and large accomplishments. Small achievements can be as simple as having sustained energy throughout the day and being able to get all your errands done efficiently due to your new nutritious lifestyle. Big achievements might be waking up and feeling good about yourself. What is important is that you pat yourself on the back for trying your best to stay committed – and forgive yourself and move on when you have a blip. Focusing on the positive creates a domino effect, and soon positive results come pouring in.

Mind Reading

Mind reading is another cognitive distortion you need be wary of. Mind reading is assuming that you know what others are thinking, especially their perceptions about you. This kind of thinking is actually helpful when we need to decipher another person's body language or read between the lines. However, extreme doses of mind reading can be problematic.

When they catch people looking at them, mind readers assume the worst and that others are developing a negative opinion about them. For example, when someone appears to be bored in a conversation with them, mind readers might assume that the other person thinks they are stupid and incompetent. Without any additional evidence, mind readers make conclusions about other people and, ultimately, about themselves. These conclusions are typically negative and unfounded, and also serve to make you unhappy. This type of distorted thinking is common in people who experience 'self-stigma' – because they stigmatise themselves, they assume others are doing the same.

How to Fix Mind Reading

Before assuming the worst and reacting rashly to a situation, take a step back and collect your thoughts. Can you really predict what others are thinking and feeling? Ask yourself whether you are making assumptions about what is going on in the minds of others and whether there is enough convincing evidence to support these assumptions. Often, you will realise that the negative thoughts are only coming from your own mind.

It's good practice to say your assumptions out loud to yourself or to write them down to hear or see your explanation in your own words. It becomes easier to see how illogical some of your assumptions are. However, if you ever discover that others do have an unfavourable opinion of you, be careful not to allow mind reading to escalate into allowing the negativity of others to validate your poor self-worth. The negative impressions of other people say less about you and more about them. It might mean there are some expectations you cannot meet, and should not try to meet.

Catastrophising

Catastrophising is assuming things to be far worse than they actually are. It involves putting a 'negative spin' on various events, compelling you to make rash and untimely decisions.[6] Catastrophising is creating fears and situations that have not yet happened, which can seriously limit the opportunities in your relationships, at work and in life – including in your efforts to beat obesity.

As with black and white thinking, one small lapse in your efforts is taken as a sign of utter and complete failure and leads to the conclusion that there is no hope of ever achieving your goals. This type of thinking can create a self-fulfilling prophecy of underachievement and disappointment. It becomes the breeding ground for overly dramatic reactions that are disproportionate to the real impact of a negative situation, or even just a negative idea. It's striking out even before getting to the plate.

There is also the possibility of over-generalising one small setback in one area of your life and convincing yourself that it holds true for all other parts. For instance, there are many possible explanations for why romantic relationships end, but an obese person who likes to mentally catastrophise may think that it's because of their weight or their difficulty losing weight. They assume that they will never meet anyone who will accept them, and therefore there is no point in even trying to change. All hope is lost from the perspective of people who think this way, believing that future prospects are worthless and that trying is fruitless. It is a mental paralysis that prevents you from taking action towards becoming the person you want to be and doing the things you want to do. Catastrophising provides you with justification for staying as you are rather than learning to take better care of yourself.

How to Fix a Catastrophising Mentality

As a famous quote from baseball legend Babe Ruth goes, 'Never let the fear of striking out keep you from playing the game.' Instead of reacting, recognise your fears and become comfortable accommodating them into your mind. This helps you move from being immobilised by fears to understanding where they are coming from. When you have a better understanding of your thinking habits, you begin to see the pattern of catastrophising.

Mental pattern recognition can be carried out in conjunction with your journalling and mood diaries, which were discussed in the previous chapter on emotional well-being. Write down the details of the event that triggered your spree of negative thoughts. Be as detailed about the event as possible and include your thoughts on the event, what your options were and what behaviour you chose.

When negativity begins to spiral, you can learn to talk back to your negative thoughts and counter their claims to take back control. This takes a lot of practice, conscious effort and mindfulness during various situations, but it can begin to reduce the frequency of catastrophising.[7]

When you are confronted with a minor difficulty – forgetting the key ingredient to a meal you were planning for this evening, having an argument with a friend or missing your train – compartmentalise it. These are setbacks in one aspect of your life and don't define your entire life. More importantly, these are setbacks that you can come back from.

Self-Criticism

Self-criticism is about how you evaluate yourself, and is characterised by excessively focusing on the areas that are a source of discontent – which ends up disqualifying or downplaying the many positive moments or achievements in your life. Commonly, it leads to name calling and general putdowns – 'You idiot!' or 'You are so greedy!'

Excessively criticising yourself means you constantly feel bad about yourself – who you are, the way you look, the choices you make. It is by far one of the most detrimental ways of thinking when it comes to beating obesity. Why? Because it leads to self-hate – and if you don't like yourself, why adopt a lifestyle that will make you healthier and happier? Why be kind to yourself?

How to Fix Self-Criticism

Instead of being too hard on yourself, treat yourself with kindness. Identify the areas where there might be room for improvement, but don't fixate on them to the point that you neglect all the other wonderful things that life (and you) has to offer.

One of the factors that fuels negative self-criticism is having a poor sense of self-identify. Some people who have struggled with obesity for a long time can start to associate their identity with their weight, and imagining themselves any other way creates an unsettling thought. If you have trouble with this, it's important to learn the second habit in Stephen Covey's world-renowned book *The 7 Habits of Highly Effective People*: 'Begin with the end in mind.'[8]

Feeling confident about a better, more positive and healthier self-image is a good start towards achieving success and owning it. An effective tool to inspire and help you imagine a healthier you is using a vision board where you can cut out and paste images, printed words and quotes that remind you of your goals and help keep you motivated. This can pave the way towards building a more positive self-identity.

Reflecting on negative thoughts and self-beliefs as they arise is another beneficial exercise for disempowering self-critical thoughts. Ask yourself the following questions whenever you have a self-critical thought:

- What are the benefits of believing this thought (e.g. added motivation and protection from bad outcomes)?

- What are the costs of believing this thought (e.g. self-consciousness, anxiety and constant fear)?

- Is the price of this negative self-belief worth my time and energy?

The health coach Jamie Mendell suggests categorising your thoughts as either coming from your inner critic (your ego) or your inner, true self (your rational, self-compassionate self).[9] She also suggests defining and embracing a true self that is happy and loving, which is a stark contrast to the inner critic that is negative, always on the attack, and doesn't understand what it means to be happy. This helps segregate the self-building thoughts from the illogical, self-defeating ones.

When it comes to cognitive well-being, often the only thing standing between you and your success is yourself. When cognitive distortions come up, the best form of defence is to be kind, compassionate and supportive to yourself.

Over to You!

Negative mental thinking can only stand in the way of beating obesity if you allow it to. If you choose to take charge, talk back to the negative ideas your inner critic makes, and adopt a more flexible frame of mind, there is no stopping you from becoming the healthy person you envision yourself to be. Take a look at the questions below and take some time to reflect on each of them.

✎ **What is the style of your dietary intake? Do you classify certain foods as completely good or bad? How does that affect your dietary decision making and the way you feel about yourself and food?**

_____

_____

_____

_____

_____

_____

_____

✎ What thoughts enter your mind when you speak with another person who seems disinterested? What could a counter-argument be to your assumption?

Assumption: _____

_____

_____

_____

_____

_____

Counter-argument: _____

_____

_____

_____

_____

_____

✎ Imagine yourself giving in to a brief overeating episode or skipping some physical activity you had planned. What would your inner critic say? Now, what would your true self say?

Inner critic: _____

_____

_____

_____

_____

_____

True self: _____

_____

_____

_____

_____

_____

In this chapter, you have gained a better understanding of how to identify the negative mental distortions that prevent you from moving towards a healthier you. The key message is to be your own best friend, not your own worst enemy.

Now that you are more prepared to control your thinking patterns, it is time to take a look at your behavioural well-being in relation to beating obesity.

· Chapter 10

Your Behavioural Well-Being

> " *If you always do what you've always done, you'll always get what you've always got.* "
>
> Henry Ford

You might be surprised at just how much your habits are getting in the way of beating obesity. The good news is that habits are within your power to change. Also, just as habits can be bad for you, you can use them to your advantage by creating new, healthier habits.

What Are Habits?

Habits are the things we do without thinking because we have done them so often in the past that they have become automatic and routine for us, like brushing our teeth. Interestingly, about 40% of all our daily tasks are habits.[1] In this way, habits are beneficial because they prevent us from having to exert too much energy on routine activities. Instead, our brains can focus on learning new tasks and solving new problems.

The problem is when bad habits have been formed – and bad habits can sneak in so easily. It all starts out so innocently. A colleague brings in doughnuts one Friday afternoon. The next week, you pass a cake shop and think maybe you should reciprocate. Before you know it, you have an unspoken agreement with your colleague that Friday is doughnut day. Of course, the odd doughnut doesn't hurt, but what about the habit recently formed at home now that your in-laws come every weekend with a bottle of wine and a box of chocolates? Or your habit of sitting in front of the TV every evening?

Habits are so easy to form and yet so hard to break. So turn this to your advantage by forming healthy habits! In the above example, if Friday must be a day of treats for you and your colleague, spice things up with some surprise healthy treats. Who can find the most delicious healthy treat? Even better, who can *make* the most delicious healthy treat? In order to replace a bad habit, the new habit needs to have some reward — such as being fun and pleasurable, or making us happy.

Eating Habits

The habits that can get in the way of beating obesity tend to be eating habits. Listed in the table below are some eating habits, what the research says about those habits, the feelings and thoughts that usually accompany them, and suggested solutions for you to break free from those behaviours.

Habit	Explanation	Associated thoughts	Solution
Buying processed snack foods in bulk and stocking up the cupboards with processed snack foods	Supermarkets where cheap food can be bought in bulk have resulted in people buying more food than they can eat.[a] The problem is, when there is more food available and accessible, some people have problems with self-control. Their appetites and desire to eat expand with the amount of food readily available.	'I save money if I buy food in bulk.' 'I need to have food in the house in case guests drop by or I feel like eating.' 'Buying in bulk saves me time having to shop every day.'	Buy fruits and vegetables, lean meats, grains and nuts in bulk. That way, when you feel like snacking, you can snack on healthy food. Buy snack items in smaller containers and smaller quantities.

Habit	Explanation	Associated thoughts	Solution
Snacking when sleepy, or eating to stay alert	People who don't get adequate amounts of night-time sleep have a greater appetite during the day.[b] This is because lack of night-time sleep lowers the metabolism of the body, causing the secretion of the stress hormone cortisol, which increases appetite.	'I feel so low in energy – I must be hungry.' 'I feel so sleepy, but I can't take a nap right now, I have a report to do. Some sugar will liven me up.'	Prioritise getting enough sleep. Drink a glass of water, do some stretching, walk around a bit and then go back to work. Wash your face with cold water. If possible, take a short nap. You'll feel more refreshed when you wake up.
Eating fast food	Fast food establishments use a lot of red and yellow colours in their decor because these colours enhance the appetite; not only do you end up buying fatty food, you also tend to eat more of it.[c]	'I don't know what to cook, so I think I'll just grab a burger and fries.' 'I don't really feel like fixing myself a meal, so why don't I grab a takeaway on the way home?' 'I'm in a rush; takeaway will be quicker.'	Drink a glass of water before you eat. Order a side salad to help fill you up. Order a child's meal if you know you will be eating later.
Eating while watching TV, reading, or surfing the web	This is also known as 'eating amnesia'.[d] What happens is you're not paying attention to what you are eating or how much you are eating. We have all done this. We have just sat down to watch our favourite TV programme with a packet of biscuits, only to find we somehow managed to finish the whole packet.	'I am all alone and don't have anybody to talk to while I eat; I might as well entertain myself and watch TV.' 'Why don't I multitask? Check my email and eat at the same time? I can save time that way.'	Eat in a room with no gadgets so that you don't get tempted – somewhere with a window so you can watch the world instead. Focus on your meal, enjoying every bite of it. You will learn more about mindful eating in Chapter 12.

Emptying our plate	The amount of food we need varies each day, so if you clear your plate every day regardless, think about whether this is merely a habit that might have been developed in childhood.	'Waste not, want not.' 'My mother would kill me if she knew I was wasting food!'	Eat slowly and chew your food completely before swallowing. If it helps, put your utensils down between each mouthful. Stop when you feel full, even if there's still more on your plate. We will be exploring how to identify hunger and fullness in Chapter 12.

a Bushak, L. (2015) 'Cheap food, more Wal-Marts contribute to rising obesity rates: How the economy is making you fat.' Medical Daily. Available at www.medicaldaily.com/cheap-food-more-wal-marts-contribute-rising-obesity-rates-how-economy-making-you-fat-320284 (accessed 11 July 2016).

b Ratini, M. (2014) 'Sleep more, weigh less.' WebMD Diet and Weight Management. Available at www.webmd.com/diet/sleep-and-weight-loss (accessed 11 July 2016).

c Dupont, A.M. (2014) 'An examination of chain restaurants exterior colors and logo colors.' University of New Hampshire Scholars' Repository, Honors Theses Paper 169. Available at http://scholars.unh.edu/cgi/viewcontent.cgi?article=1170&context=honors (accessed 16 July 2016).

d Davis, J.L. (2007) 'Top 10 bad habits that lead to weight gain.' WebMD Weight Loss and Obesity Feature Archive. Available at www.webmd.com/diet/obesity/top-10-bad-habits-that-lead-to-weight-gain (accessed 11 July 2016).

How Can I Break a Bad Habit?

To change a habit, you must first recognise the behaviour as a habit. This can be difficult: by their very nature, habits are automatic and not easily detectable – they are just the way we do things. However, once you identify a habit, you can then look at the structure of that habit by asking yourself:

- What are the triggers of the habit I want to change?

- What are the actions included in this habit?

- What reward do I get from this repeated action?

- How can I replace that reward to ensure that I don't feel the need to return to that particular habit?

Once you have figured out which bad habits need changing, you can derail the habits by creating windows of opportunity to act on new intentions. This means identifying the external triggers that influence you. For example, if you tend to eat more while watching emotional TV programmes, it would be good to change your viewing – or, even better, to have the TV off when you are eating.

Unhealthy habits are easier to remove if you replace them. Furthermore, healthy behaviours will not become habits unless they are repeated over time and result in some kind of reward – even if that reward is a sense of achievement at choosing a healthy behaviour over an unhealthy alternative.

Nudge Yourself Towards Healthier Habits

The UK is the first country to use some of the principles of Nudge Theory as part of government policy to decrease the percentage of obese and overweight adults.[2] The government did this by increasing incentives for manufacturers to market food (especially junk food) in smaller packages. The theory is, if the packages are smaller, people will tend to eat less.

In a nutshell, Nudge Theory, when applied to health, involves slightly changing the environment to help people make voluntary decisions that are healthier and that they usually want to make but find difficult. For instance, if you would like to eat more fruit and less junk food each day, you can put the fruit in a more accessible place (e.g. on the kitchen counter) and the junk food on the topmost shelf. These are simple yet effective techniques to help you adopt healthier behaviours, because humans are designed to conserve energy and go for the easier option.

If you would like to drink more water and fewer fizzy drinks, put a bottle of water on your desk or wherever you spend most of your time. You will find that you are much more likely to reach for this when you are thirsty than seek out another option.

In both examples above, you still have an option. The junk food is there, and so is the fizzy drink. So you don't feel 'deprived' of the foods and drinks that you have been accustomed to because you still have the choice to eat or drink them. Your choices haven't been limited by anyone, but making them the more difficult option will help the healthier options become your new 'default'.

Over to You!

Many of the habits discussed in this chapter are automatic and experienced by most people to a lesser or greater degree. Ask yourself now:

✎ **What habits do I have that defeat my efforts to be healthier? These can be habits not listed above.**

_____

_____

_____

_____

_____

_____

_____

_____

✎ **Why are these habits so hard to break? What reward are they giving me?**

_____

_____

_____

_____

_____

_____

_____

_____

✎ **What healthier habits could replace the habits identified above and provide me with a similar reward?**

Unhealthy habit	Healthy habit replacement

Habits can be closely linked to relationships, such as carrying out the same unhealthy behaviours with a particular friend. Let's take a look at how you can work on your relationships and social well-being to ensure these don't hinder your efforts to reach your health goals.

Chapter 11

Your Social Well-Being

> " *No road is long with good company.*
>
> Turkish Proverb "

According to Dr Nicole Avena, author of *Why Diets Fail,* research into addiction recovery has shown that social relationships are almost indispensable when it comes to success in beating addiction, including addiction to food.[1] Indeed, one study examining multiple factors that affected the maintenance of weight in people who had undergone bariatric surgery found that those with strong emotional and social support networks were most likely to be able to keep the weight off.[2]

This study also found that those who were able to understand that they were using food as an emotional regulator and were able to detach their emotions from their eating habits were more successful in maintaining their weight. This suggests that harmful eating habits are closely linked to emotional states. Since your closest friends and family are the ones most likely to affect your emotional state, the importance of distancing yourself from negative influences and embracing positive ones becomes vital when working towards beating obesity.

You can divide your social support into three broad groups: emotional, practical and inspirational.

Emotional Support

Emotional support comes in the form of friends and family who offer you a shoulder to lean on when things seem insurmountable. They are able to take some of the burden off your shoulders, and just talking to them helps make you feel that your goal is not as impossible as it may seem at times. Such support is important when you are dealing with setbacks along the road to better health and well-being. Friends and family who can offer you encouragement along the way are the best people to have around.

Negative emotional influence comes from people who make you feel bad about yourself. They might not even know they are doing this and probably don't have any malicious intent, but that doesn't change the fact that it can demoralise you and derail your plans. Attempt to confront them and explain how their actions and words are impeding your progress to a healthier lifestyle. If this doesn't work, take steps to distance yourself from them. If distancing yourself isn't possible, spend as little time with them as you can, especially while you are in the early stages of your journey to beat obesity.

Many people struggling with obesity also struggle with low self-esteem and body image issues. So when others comment negatively on your weight, appearance or behaviour patterns – particularly friends and family – this will damage your self-esteem further. Developing a positive body image is important in beating obesity for the long term, so spend as little time as possible with those who make you feel bad about yourself.

A theory known as 'systems theory' can help you understand how your family affects you emotionally.[3] This theory states that everyone in a family is intensely emotionally connected and that the interactions between family members have complex and far-reaching consequences. For example, if one member of your family gets anxious, then this anxiety can spread quickly and intensify among everyone else. Therefore, it is in the best interests of everyone to help each other. Of course, this is an ideal that isn't achievable for everyone. Indeed, it is important to highlight here that if you lack family support, this doesn't mean you are doomed. Far from it. You can beat obesity without their support. It might just take a greater level of will and motivation on your part. But what a sense of achievement will come from that!

Ask yourself the following questions to identify the best and worst sources of emotional support around you:

- Are my weight problems associated with the comments or actions of others during my childhood or adolescence?

- Does anyone around me constantly criticise me?

- Who has offered me positive encouragement and praise for my previous achievements?

- Who seems the happiest and most secure around me?

- Who tries to help me with my lifestyle goals?

- Does anyone try to hinder my goals by putting obstacles in my way?

Answering these questions will help you establish the people in your life who are supporters rather than criticisers. You are then equipped to decide whether you would like to spend more or less time with the various people in your social world.

Practical Support

Practical support refers to the people who will guide you through the day-to-day tasks that will help you beat obesity. For example, a friend or family member might offer to look after your kids while you go for a walk, or your boss may offer you a company-paid gym membership. The most important thing to remember when it comes to receiving practical support is that you won't necessarily get it if you don't ask for it. Even your closest friends with the best intentions might not be able to guess what practical help will assist you the most. So, start as you mean to go on, making your intentions to beat obesity public to those whom you trust to be supportive. This will alert significant people in your life that you are embarking on a challenging journey and might need their help. Make sure that you are clear about what you need from them.

Negative practical support comes from those around you who put obstacles in your way. You may have a colleague, for example, who regularly brings in cakes to work and insists that you have one as a reward for doing so well with your lifestyle plan. Such people frequently place temptation in front of you. If they continue to do so even after you explain to them that you are trying to be healthier and kinder to yourself, try to keep your distance from them. You have done your part by informing them, and there is nothing impolite about refusing to indulge in behaviour that is detrimental to your health and well-being. If you value these relationships for other reasons, you can suggest alternative activities so that you still spend time with them.

Inspirational Support

Inspirational support comes from people around you who motivate and encourage you to achieve your goals. The most useful and common tool from which to draw inspirational support is through vicarious experiences (knowledge gained through observing others), as discussed in Chapter 6 on how to boost your confidence. Find forums online or offline (such as Weight Watchers) where people share their own stories of goal achievement, especially in terms of beating obesity.

You can also seek help from family and friends who have overcome other obstacles. Even if they didn't have a problem with obesity, most people have dealt with a difficult issue and can use their experience to teach you a few things about how to approach your own problem.

Seeking inspiration from success stories is a great way to get yourself out of the house and be social. However, if you find yourself without the will or energy to step out, find an article, blog post or video that will help you find some inspiration. Talking to an encouraging friend will also be useful.

Friends who have similar problems to your own but aren't actively trying to fight these problems will influence you negatively, however. If your friendship revolves around shared bad habits like binge eating or drinking too much alcohol, you might want to consider ways to ensure they don't jeopardise your plans for a healthier lifestyle. You might even want to share your journey with them and provide them with the opportunity to join you on the road towards a healthier lifestyle. At the end of the day, the choices these friends make are not up to you, and if their choices are affecting your journey, you may need to choose between them and your health.

Think back to the stages of behaviour change discussed in Chapter 5. If you are in the action stage and your friend is in the pre-contemplation stage, the relationship could harm your progress. Alternatively, you might end up being the inspiration for your friend to enter the contemplation stage. When assessing whether a friendship is helpful or harmful to your own health, be honest with yourself.

Embracing Your Friends

To get the most out of your support network, it is worth considering changing the way you interact with those who are supporting you the most:

- **Don't let guilt or shame get in the way of making contact.** If you have a slip-up and are too ashamed to admit it to your friends, then you are unlikely to get the support you need.

- **Remember that relationships go both ways.** Make sure you don't keep imposing on your friends for support without offering support back. Remember that everyone is facing stress or struggles of some kind. Do you best to return the help.

- **Select roles for your support network carefully.** Different people around you will be able to offer you support in various ways. Choose who is best at providing emotional, practical and inspirational support. Your work colleague may not be the best person to listen to your problems and offer emotional support, but they may be able to offer company for a regular lunchtime walk.

Seeking Professional Support

If you think that your closest friends or family may not be able to help you on your journey, it might be better to look elsewhere. Fortunately, there are many resources available to those who want to beat obesity. Your doctor, a counsellor or a nutritionist are great resources to offer you one-to-one advice and expert opinion. Don't be shy to ask questions and invite ideas when you need them. These people can also direct you to other resources so that you can form a strong support network around you.

There are different types of counselling to choose from, the following three being particularly useful for beating obesity:

- **Cognitive behavioural counselling.** You learn how to create and maintain positive habits and ways to 'unlearn' bad habits and replace them with more wholesome ones. This type of counselling will help you change the thoughts that impact your behaviour. If you found Chapter 9 on cognitive well-being particularly relevant and useful, then this might be the best form of counselling for you.

- **Person-centred counselling.** Here, you learn about the value of being open to life, as well as about the healing power of unconditional acceptance of yourself and others. This type of counselling provides an accepting and non-judgemental space for you to explore your thoughts and feelings and develop your self-belief. If you found

Chapter 6 on confidence tapped into a need to work on your self-belief, then this might be the best form of counselling for you.

- **Psychodynamic counselling.** You learn to discover the hidden meanings behind your fears, fantasies, emotions and behaviours. This type of counselling is most appropriate if you feel your problems are related to childhood experiences and you feel ready to explore these experiences in a supportive environment. If you found Chapter 8 on your emotional well-being highlighted areas you need to work on, then this might be the best form of counselling for you.

Whichever type of counselling you choose, you can expect the following:

- **You, the client.** You will do most of the talking, but your counsellor might ask some questions to get a better understanding of your problems. It might be difficult at first, but if you are open, honest and committed, you can benefit from counselling.

- **The counsellor.** A counsellor will offer you a relaxed, safe environment of support, encouragement and hope. They will help you to express your thoughts and feelings without fear of judgement.

Here are some of the ways in which seeing a counsellor could help you:

- **Relief of symptoms.** Speaking to someone who cares can bring relief of symptoms related to obesity, whether they are physical or emotional

- **Trust, emotional support and encouragement.** Finding someone you can trust isn't always easy, but you can trust your counsellor.

- **Boost in confidence and self-esteem.** Counselling helps you find your own solutions to your problems.

- **Learning new skills.** How to deal with urges to comfort eat, how to motivate yourself to be more active and how to be mindful are just some of the skills you can learn in counselling.

- **Sense of control.** Counselling can help you gain control over the choices you make related to your health and well-being.

- **Greater fulfilment.** As you begin to better manage any daily or stressful challenges related to your efforts to beat obesity, you begin to live more creatively and experience life and its challenges with more ease, acceptance and fulfilment.

Over to You!

✎ **Who is in my support network?**

I can rely on the following people for emotional support	I can rely on the following people for practical support	I can rely on the following people for inspirational support

✎ Could I benefit from counselling? Tick all that apply:

☐ I use food to cope with my emotions.

☐ My weight problems are related to my childhood.

☐ I feel out of control.

☐ I struggle with low mood and/or anxiety.

☐ I hate myself.

☐ I lack confidence.

☐ I have no one to talk to about my problems.

☐ I just don't know how to cope.

Everyone could benefit from counselling, but the more boxes you ticked, the more likely counselling will help you.

Now that you have the tools and network in place to cope with the challenges of beating obesity, let's move on to your dietary well-being.

Chapter 12

Your Dietary Well-Being

> *The doctor of the future will no longer treat the human frame with drugs, but rather will cure and prevent disease with nutrition.*
>
> Thomas Edison

Beating obesity will certainly entail making smarter dietary decisions and eating less of certain types of food, but as mentioned in Chapter 3 (Why Beat Obesity?), eating too little to the point that your body goes into starvation mode (which slows down your metabolism) isn't going to help with achieving your goals.

According to Sandra Aamodt, neuroscientist and author of *Why Diets Make Us Fat*, the human body has a set point or a set minimum range of weight levels that it aims to maintain.[1] Set points vary from person to person. That means our bodies may have a threshold for weight loss. Interestingly, no matter how much dieting and exercise we push our bodies to withstand, our body will eventually revert to its set point. Often, some people pressure themselves to achieve weight levels that are way below their set point, which leads to years of yo-yo dieting and a constant sense of dissatisfaction with their body.

This isn't to be taken as a sign that there is no point in adjusting your diet. On the contrary, adjusting your diet teaches you to become more familiar with your own body in order to begin to understand that your nutritional needs may not be the same as those of the person sitting next to you. More importantly, adjusting your diet teaches you that dietary well-being does not constitute avoiding food and losing as much weight as possible to look like somebody else; instead, it is about building a healthy perspective and healthy behaviours around food choices that suit you and your lifestyle.

Changing Your Idea of 'Dieting'

In the previous chapters, the importance of emotional, social and cognitive well-being in beating obesity were discussed. At this point, it should be clearer that overcoming obesity is actually less about weight loss and more about self-care.

Dieting should also be seen in the same light – as a way for you to take care of yourself. Once you see food for what it is – as a source of energy – you can begin to nurture a more positive relationship with food.

Making healthier food choices should not be a struggle, but the word 'diet' has been used so lightly and so often that for many people it has come to mean restraining yourself from enjoying food or even consuming food. Being thin as a result of food restriction can mean being undernourished, whereas being healthy means your body receives all the essential nutrients it needs to function optimally. Health needs to be your goal; your optimal weight will follow.

Addictive Behaviours

Food addictions and comfort eating can complicate your dietary decision making. The urge to eat is a difficult thing to stop for most people, whether they struggle with their weight or not. Typically, the addiction is for junk foods, which tend to be extremely high in salt, sugar or bad fat.

Junk Food and Addiction

Eating too much junk food too often triggers the reward and pleasure centres of the brain by releasing the feel-good neurotransmitter dopamine (a chemical in the brain). This hormone is so powerful that, for susceptible people, eating junk food can lead to addiction. This pleasure system in our brain was originally designed to reward us in ways that encouraged survival, but the junk foods of today release excessive amounts of this feel-good chemical.

By repeatedly doing something that releases dopamine in the reward system, such as eating chocolate, the brain starts to remove the excessive dopamine receptors in order to restore balance. However, with fewer receptors, more dopamine is needed to reach the same level of pleasure. Ultimately, increasing amounts of junk food are required to achieve feelings of pleasure that could once be derived from much less junk food. In other words, you have built up a tolerance to junk food.

The impact of junk food addiction isn't unlike being addicted to drugs, and people with junk food addiction will even experience withdrawal if they don't get a junk food 'fix'. Junk foods become 'trigger' foods that perpetuate a cycle of craving, hunger, overeating and guilt.[2] David Kessler, a former commissioner of the Food and Drug Administration (FDA) and author of the book *The End of Overeating*, has even accused food manufacturers of manipulating the sugar, salt and fat levels of foods to feed an addiction at the neurochemical level.[3]

Junk Food and the Gut

Junk food can also change your gut in a way that makes it difficult to manage your weight. Indeed, some researchers have looked into the possibility that sugary and salty foods can alter the normal composition of the microbes in the human intestines. Studies have found that certain bacteria in the gut have the ability to induce hunger and insulin resistance in rodents, suggesting the same could be true with humans.[4] The problem arises when junk food becomes the staple diet. The high salt, high fat and high sugar content in the junk food activates the microbes to signal the brain to eat more food.

Overcoming Food Addiction

In the hopes of reducing the consumption of foods high in sugar, some health experts are lobbying to tax sugar, just as governments would with other highly addicting substances such as alcohol and tobacco.[5] In the UK, a new sugar tax on soft drinks is set to be introduced, while Norway already taxes chocolate and sweets, and Finland and France tax sweetened drinks.

Overcoming food addiction, however, is also in your hands. You must first be able to identify which foods are junk for the body. If you can manage to minimise your exposure to foods that trigger your cravings, then you will feel more in control of choosing healthier food options. This will help you begin to visualise what a balanced and nutritious diet looks like.

Sugary soft drinks and other unhealthy food items that may be a normal part of your old lifestyle will need to play a much smaller role in your life, so it is important that you find a way to cleanse your palate of the flavour of sugar, salt and fat. There may be no need to completely eradicate these foods, but for the sake of your dietary well-being, you will need to cut down on these foods or look for healthier alternatives.

A Nutrition-Oriented Perspective

Studies have found that people who previously struggled with being overweight, but are then able to maintain their healthier weight, share common behaviours:

- They start to prefer eating naturally healthy foods that are low in sugar, salt or fat.

- They also develop and stick to a diet that is based on their own body's needs and their individual goals and lifestyle, rather than strictly following a fad diet suited to someone else's lifestyle.[6]

Whichever food types you may prefer, what is universal is that there is only one right approach to making dietary decisions: a nutrition-based one. So what exactly does a nutrition-based diet look like?

According to the new Eatwell Guide, developed by Public Health England (PHE), people must include more fruits, vegetables and wholegrain starchy carbohydrates in their diets to meet the body's nutrient requirements. Specifically, a healthy and balanced diet comprises:[7]

- at least five portions of various fruits and vegetables a day

- basing meals on starchy carbohydrates such as potatoes, bread, rice or pasta (ideally wholegrain)

- including some dairy or dairy alternatives (such us soya drinks) in your diet (preferably lower fat and sugar options)

- eating some beans, pulses, fish, eggs, meat and other proteins (including two portions of fish every week, one of which should be oily)

- opting for unsaturated oils and spreads and consuming them in small amounts.

In addition, the six basic nutrients you require for good health are:

- carbohydrate

- protein

- fat

- minerals

- vitamins

- water.

The table below provides more details on these six basic nutrients.

Nutrient	Source
Carbohydrate	**Simple carbohydrates** are simply sugars, as found in chocolate, ice cream, cake, etc. A small amount of this is fine, but the carbohydrates you really want are **complex carbohydrates** – starch plus soluble fibre. Good sources are fruits, vegetables, nuts, seeds, brown rice, oats, barley and rice bran.
Protein	Good sources of **plant-based proteins** are soybeans, nuts and legumes. Good sources of **animal-based proteins** are lean meats and fish.
Fat	Good fats are olive and canola oils and avocados.
Minerals	**Calcium** – This helps keep teeth and bones strong and healthy. Good sources are tofu, low-fat cheese, yogurt and milk. **Iron** – For building muscles and keeping blood healthy. Good sources are pumpkin seeds, spinach, soybeans and lentils, as well as liver and oysters. **Zinc** – This helps build a healthy immune system and also helps with fertility. It can be found in dark chocolate, spinach, beans and cashew nuts. **Magnesium** – Helps the proper functioning of nerves and muscles. It also neutralises stomach acids and helps move food along the digestive tract. Good sources include milk, lean meats, seeds and nuts.

Vitamins	**A** – This vitamin keeps skin, eyes and teeth healthy. It can be found in carrots, sweet potatoes, cantaloupe and other orange-coloured fruits and vegetables.
	B – There are eight B vitamins, all of which play a unique role in energy production. To ensure you are getting a mixture of these eight vitamins, include a variety of whole grains, fruits and vegetables in your diet. For Vitamin B12, however, you will also need animal sources, such as milk, yoghurt and egg yolks.
	C – This vitamin helps to strengthen blood vessels and maintain elasticity of the skin. Good sources are guavas, citrus fruits such as oranges and grapefruits, cantaloupe and red and green peppers.
	D – For strong bones. Can be found in eggs, fish and mushrooms.
	E – Helps blood circulation. Can be found in almonds, tomatoes, sunflower seeds and nuts.
	K – This vitamin helps blood to clot. Good sources are dark green leafy vegetables such as kale, spinach, Brussels sprouts and broccoli.
	Folic acid – This helps in cell renewal and prevents birth defects. It can be found in peas, beans, cauliflower, beets, asparagus, lentils, seeds and nuts.
Water	Water is required for most bodily functions as it maintains the health of every cell in the body. You don't need to get water simply from drinking the liquid format. You can also find it in most foods, especially fruits. However, the body can only get about 20% of its total water from solid foods alone. You ideally need 6–8 glasses of water daily.[a]

a Public Health England 2016.

If you feel the need to consume foods or drinks that are high in sugar, fat or salt – especially at the beginning of your journey to beat obesity – eat or drink them in small amounts and less often. Additionally, try to drink plenty of water. It isn't a myth that we can mistake thirst for hunger.

Essentially, by having a nutrition-based approach to choosing the mix of foods you take in, you can better understand the nutritional role of food in the body and start to nurture a healthier relationship with food. The end goal of knowing about the nutritional facts of each food type is to empower you to create the dietary balance that you are comfortable with and can commit to.

If you still aren't sure how all of this translates into your daily lifestyle, the Eatwell Guide below can be a useful benchmark for assessing if you are on the right track:

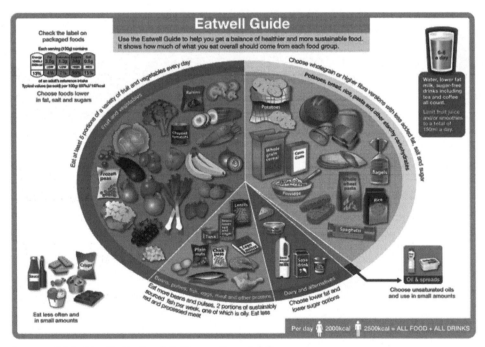

Source: Public Health England © Crown Copyright[8]

Foods for Beating Obesity

Beating obesity is about a healthy and nutritious lifestyle rather than any specific foods, but there are some foods that can help you along the way:[9]

- Whole grains such as barley, corn, oats, rice and rye are complex carbohydrates that aren't easily broken down into sugar because they have a lot of soluble fibre. They give you energy for physical activity.

- Vegetables and fruits have vitamins and minerals that help regulate your body's processes. They help to keep you feeling full for longer periods of time. The sugars in fruit help satisfy cravings for sweets.

- Nuts, seeds and lean meats have protein to help you build muscle mass; muscle burns more energy than fat, helping you to balance energy input and output.

Using a Food Diary

Using a food diary is an effective way of keeping on track with your lifestyle goals. It also helps you establish problem areas where you might need greater support or more resolve. Monitoring your hunger and fullness levels is also highly beneficial in terms of controlling food, rather than food controlling you.

The table below is adapted from Bates College Health Centre.[10] By using this, you can monitor your hunger levels and become more mindful of how you assess and address your hunger cues.

Location, date and time	Hunger level before eating	Description of food and drink consumed	Fullness level after eating	Thoughts and feelings	Possible triggor

The hunger and fullness levels can be scored based on the Hunger Scale shown on the next page.

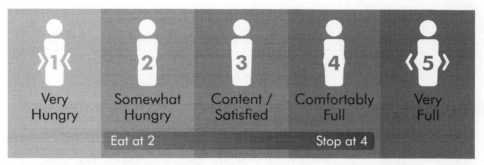

Source: Nourish Move Thrive[11]

This scale can also help you identify when to eat and when to stop eating. It can be dangerous to eat when in the 'Very Hungry' range as this is a recipe for overeating, so always try to eat when you are 'Somewhat Hungry' and before you become ravenous.

As discussed in previous chapters, tracking your thoughts and feelings can help you to examine and improve your emotional, social and cognitive well-being. The same is true for your dietary well-being. Tracking your thoughts and feelings can help you to identify the possible triggers of your eating impulses, which could include specific food items, food cravings, being surrounded by food establishments, seeing something on television or being with friends who love to eat. These are root causes that you can learn to recognise and manage.

Mindful Eating and Intelligent Eating

While nutrition is about *what* to eat, mindful eating is about *how* you eat. It is directing your full attention to the experience of eating while practising appreciation, respect and enjoyment for the food that is available to you. This practice can help you on your journey towards health.[12]

Mindful eating is about how focusing on a food's flavour, colour, texture and consistency stimulates your senses, rather than eating food without thought or reflection. It is based on the idea that you have the power to be conscious about what you eat and why you eat by basing your eating on the body's physical cue for hunger, rather than on emotional cues. In one interview, the neuroscientist Sandra Aamodt defined mindful eating as eating with attention and joy, and without judgement, including attention to feelings of hunger and fullness.[13]

Carolyn Ross, an eating disorder and addictions expert, emphasises that mindful eating should not be mistaken as a form of dieting; rather, it is an exercise in reconnecting with your body's needs. It is about recognising the hunger and fullness signals of the body and experiencing the taste, smell, texture and visual image of the food.[14] Some people who struggle with managing their food intake worry that savouring their food will lead to overeating, but it tends to have the opposite effects as you are left feeling more satisfied by the experience. You have also eaten more slowly, giving your body time to digest the food and signal to your brain that you are full.[15]

A term related to mindful eating is intelligent eating, also known as intuitive eating. Intelligent eating is about empowering yourself through information and knowledge, so that you can make smart dietary choices and ultimately take control of your health.[16] It is also about developing a relationship with food that is characterised by eating for physical instead of emotional reasons, relying on internal hunger cues when deciding to eat, and stopping eating when the body signals fullness. Intelligent eaters give themselves unconditional permission to eat and accept it as a normal and necessary process.

Like mindful eating, intelligent eating is helpful in beating obesity because it slows you down as you eat. When you slow down, you eat less. You eat only when you are truly hungry, instead of eating out of boredom or for other emotional reasons. When you pay full attention to what you are eating, you eat less because your brain feels satisfied with the eating experience, even when you have consumed less than you are used to eating.

People who practise mindful and intelligent eating often find themselves having a growing interest in preparing their own food or even growing their own food.

Over to You!

✎ **How aware or conscious do you think you are when you choose what food to eat, how much to eat and when to eat?**

_____

_____

_____

_____

✎ Looking back at the most recent time you found yourself eating more than your body needed, what behaviours, situations, time of the day, kind of company or other conditions were possible triggers to your eating behaviour?

_____

_____

_____

_____

_____

✎ Challenge yourself to some mindful eating. With your next meal or snack, carry out the following exercise.

Before you begin to put food in your mouth, just observe it and ask yourself:

- What appeals to my eyes about this food? Consider shape, colour and anything else that appeals.

- Why is this food before me? Is it because I have eaten it before, because I wanted something savoury or is there another reason?

- What specific tastes appeal to me about this particular food?

- What benefit will this particular food give my body?

Place the food closer to your nose.

- What appeals to my nose about this food?

Place a small piece of the food in your mouth. Don't chew it, but roll it around with your tongue, really experiencing the feel of the food against your palate.

- What is the texture like?

- How does this food feel in my mouth?

- What flavours are coming through before I have even chewed the food?

Bite the food once and ask yourself the same three questions.
   Now, welcome those flavours and finish your food with the new understanding that you have control over your food, not vice versa – and that this gives you the power to savour your food and the goodness it is supplying you with.

✎ How was this experience of mindful eating for you? Did you discover anything about yourself or about food and eating?

_____

_____

_____

_____

_____

This chapter focused on what it means to think, decide and behave from the perspective of nutrition. It is imperative to have a healthier perception of what 'dieting' means and what role food has in nourishing your body. Health comes from within, and a lack of balance in your diet can affect your nutritional needs and overall health. However, a healthy diet is best complemented by a dose of physical activity. The following chapter addresses how you can achieve physical well-being.

Chapter 13

Your Physical Well-Being

> *To keep the body in good health is a duty, otherwise we shall not be able to keep our mind strong and clear.*
>
> Buddha

Sedentary living is considered a health risk factor, especially for obese people who are prone to developing serious ailments such as diabetes and cardiovascular diseases.[1] Having some form of physical activity will help you in your journey to beat obesity and to achieve better health and well-being. Indeed, it is a myth that obese people can't be active, and in this chapter you will learn about how you can gradually introduce greater physical activity into your life.

How Much Physical Activity Is Enough?

In order to achieve a healthier weight, there is a minimum level of physical activity you will need to undertake. As discussed in Chapter 1, obesity is largely about energy in and energy out. We have explored in great detail ways to control the energy you take in, and you should be feeling more confident about this. We want to develop the same level of confidence when it comes to having better control over the energy you put out.

Spending less than 30 minutes per week doing moderate physical activity or less than 15 minutes per week doing vigorous physical activity is considered to be 'inactive'. On the other hand, spending 30–59 minutes on moderate physical activity or 15–29 minutes on vigorous physical activity comprises 'low activity'.[2]

According to the Health and Social Care Information Centre in the UK, it is recommended that adults spend at least 150 minutes per week doing moderate activity or 75 minutes per week of vigorous activity.[3] Examples of moderate activity include brisk walking, heavy housework such as hoovering or mopping, and mowing the lawn. Vigorous activity includes tennis, hiking and running.

This isn't to say that you should jump into doing 150 minutes of moderate physical activity a week. Maybe this just isn't possible for you. Remember the goal-setting exercise in Chapter 7? It applies here. Your long-term goal might be to reach the recommended level of physical activity, but your short-term goals to get there might go something like this:

- Goal 1: Be less inactive.

- Goal 2: Walk five minutes every other day for two weeks.

- Goal 3: Walk seven minutes every other day for two weeks.

- Goal 4: Walk ten minutes every other day for two weeks.

- Goal 5: Walk ten minutes every day for two weeks.

You need to go at a pace that works for you and that will help you reach your long-term goal, not put you off reaching it because it just seems too difficult. Of course, if you are already active, your goals will look very different to those above – tailor them to your current activity levels.

Overcoming Challenges with Graded Exposure

Given that diet is very effective for weight loss, why do you still need to exercise? Physical activity is more than about burning calories or cutting down body fat. Exercise also helps improve metabolism, build muscle, curb appetite, improve heart, lung and brain function, and increase mental concentration.[4]

Physical activity does come with some unique challenges for obese people, which can be limiting and frustrating;[5] they may even create a sense of fear of doing physical activity. However, there is no need to feel pressured or to over-exert yourself just to prove that you are dedicated to becoming healthier. What is needed instead is a better understanding of how to work around any limitations or fears you might have, so that you can reap the benefits of a more active lifestyle.

These benefits are less about weight loss and more about weight maintenance. Exercise plays a bigger role in weight maintenance as you start to beat obesity. In this sense, it is important to start to accept physical activity into your life while you are beating obesity in order to ensure it becomes a habit that you can maintain in order to prevent gaining weight back.

You don't have to become an athlete, however. Indeed, one study compared the effects of two treatment programmes that highlighted the importance of choosing moderate steps over aggressive actions.[6] One of the treatments aimed to reduce saturated fat intake and increase physical activity. The other treatment aimed to increase fruit and vegetable intake and reduce periods of inactivity (such as being seated for more than 30 minutes). The second treatment was found to be more effective, suggesting that making small changes to a person's sedentary lifestyle can be more effective than committing to a structured set of intense physical activities. Low-intensity exercises done regularly have also been linked to metabolic improvements and incremental weight loss.

Tips for simply being less inactive

- Use the upstairs bathroom if you are downstairs and vice versa.
- Do some stretches when brushing your teeth.
- Walk around during the adverts on TV.
- Dance while doing the housework.
- Use a small hand weight when on the phone.

Can you add any more?

Starting Simple – Walking More

Starting with walking 500 steps a day may be a more realistic and pragmatic goal than joining a gym or training for a marathon. With small achievements, you can become increasingly aware of both the limitations and possibilities of your body in terms of physical activity, which contributes towards long-term behavioural change.

Stephen Morrison, lay adviser for the Faculty of Sport and Exercise Medicine UK, was previously morbidly obese, but is now an active runner who has successfully maintained his weight loss. Fear held him back from taking part in and sustaining physical activity – fear that he would not know how to get started, that he would disappoint others or that he would fail.[7]

So, how was he able to transform into a physical activity advocate? He took small steps and more of these small steps as he gained in confidence and ability. He also became a 'try athlete' – someone who samples new sports and physical activities to find those they enjoy. Variety can help you in your efforts to be physically active, as discussed in more detail later in this chapter.

Other than keeping you healthy, walking also offers other wonders. It gets you to different places, offers different vantage points and allows you to breathe in your surroundings and have a sense of fulfilment for the distance you've covered. Walking is simple, free and non-intimidating.

Gill Stewart, Programme Director of Nordic Walking UK, encourages the use of Nordic sticks, which function very similarly to the handles of a cross trainer machine. The sticks help to pull and propel you forward, and to improve posture and tone in both arms and legs. It is an exercise for the entire body that burns up to 50% more calories than regular walking.[8]

Progressing Towards Other Exercises

As you progress on your journey to beat obesity, your metabolic rate will decrease, as described in Chapter 2. This is why exercise is so important in maintaining weight loss. Exercise is crucial in building muscle, maintaining the metabolic rate and burning fat. An additional pound of muscle burns an additional 50 calories per day, making weight loss happen faster.[9]

The objective of engaging in more physical activity is to increase your strength, stamina and flexibility, as well as to develop your muscles. The best exercises to achieve these outcomes are stretching exercises such as yoga. Yoga does not involve jumping or running, so this will be easier on your knees and ankles. Another recommended exercise for people who are obese is swimming or aqua aerobics. Carrying a lot of excess weight around can tax your muscles and joints. The water will reduce the impact of your weight on your joints and muscles when you do your exercises, and the water will also create resistance so that your muscles will stretch and work just a little bit more.

Recumbent bike is also a good exercise. It works your leg muscles as well as your core body, but the back rest of the seat will support your back muscles until they are strong enough to support your weight if you choose to move over to a regular bike.

Variety Is the Spice of Physical Activity

One of the biggest reasons for not being able to maintain a physical activity plan is boredom – for the mind and body. As being more physically active becomes a greater part of your routine, over time your body will become accustomed to it. Your muscles will have strengthened and they won't feel quite as strained as they used to. You will have reached a plateau.[10]

It is at a similar time that you might also find your mind wandering from the task at hand. Here is where variety can spice up your physical activity and keep both your mind and body on track. Rather than sticking to the same routine or activity, swap things around a bit. Maybe one day you might go for a walk, another day a swim, and another day learn a new activity that you have never tried before.

If you use a static exercise machine, such as a bike or treadmill, this can become particularly boring unless you set yourself new challenges, new times and new speeds. Also, since your environment isn't changing as you exercise on such equipment, you need to ensure you don't get bored of the view. Maybe have the TV on, or rotate the location of equipment in the house. It is also a good idea to have some music on. Do whatever it takes to keep your exercise time enjoyable. Maybe it can become the only time you listen to the radio or music, so you start to look forward to your 'me time'. You are more likely to stick to your exercise plan when you enjoy it – and you can enjoy exercise if you go about it the right way!

Ideas for adding variety to your physical activity

- Have a cleaning competition with a friend. Who can clean their house the fastest?

- Pick a sport or exercise you have never done but would like to learn.

- Change your physical activity to suit the weather. The sun has popped out? Spend the morning gardening.

- Combine exercise with something you enjoy. Love animals? A lengthy walk around the zoo can be a good workout.

- Change your treadmill pace to the different songs that come on the radio.

Can you add any more?

Overcoming Self-Consciousness

Another barrier to exercise is feeling self-conscious about your size, weight or level of fitness. This can make you feel uncomfortable about exercising where others might see you, leading to you exercising in isolation – another potential cause of boredom. Exercising in isolation is fine and might even be how you would like to start your journey to improved fitness. However, you might need extra determination to keep it up by utilising some of the tips discussed above.

It can also be worth working towards overcoming your self-consciousness, so that you have more variety available to you. Try to remind yourself that health and well-being isn't something that only certain people deserve. You deserve it too. You have every right to be healthy, and you therefore have every right to take whatever action will help you become healthy. What others think about you doesn't matter. You are not exercising for them, but to improve your own quality of life and that of any loved ones who will benefit from your lifestyle improvements.

To help beat self-consciousness, try to motivate yourself in other ways. If you want to go to use facilities at the gym or join an exercise class, treat yourself to some new exercise clothes that you feel good in. Going to learner classes can also help ease self-consciousness as everyone will be learning something new and will probably be self-conscious as well, even if it isn't for the same reason. Why not even get yourself a personal coach? They are trained to help you work to your own level of fitness and can help keep you focused on your end goal when your self-consciousness gets the better of you. You will also be so busy listening to them and working with them that you won't even notice what everyone else is up to.

Seek Support, Not Excuses

Physical activity can be a chore for many people, who often have a list of reasons that excuse them from doing even the simplest forms of exercise. Everyone is prone to this, regardless of weight. Some common excuses include the weather, the gym fee, feeling too tired, feeling uncomfortable with wearing a swimsuit or having no time.

You can come up with a thousand reasons *not* to exercise, but the key reason *to* exercise is that it is essential for health and well-being. For that reason, it can be helpful to have the right people around, who will support you through the tough times. Obesity is a complex problem, and the support and motivation of others can go a long way.

If you don't have that social support – not everyone does – don't worry. You can still do this. One way to support yourself is by redesigning your environment in a way that will make you less sedentary. Think back to Nudge Theory discussed in Chapter 10. Why not place your exercise equipment where it can't be ignored or keep your phone charger upstairs? Why not organise for a friend to knock on your door on a certain day and time for a regular walk? These are all examples of physical activity nudges that make being active easier.

The benefits of physical activity

- Increases alertness.

- Helps with critical thinking.

- Increases your sense of well-being (you've done something to make yourself healthier).

- Increases your sense of accomplishment (you've moved closer towards your health goals).

- Increases your sense of control (you set a goal and you actually did all in your power to achieve it).

- Enhances self-confidence (you did it yesterday, you did it today, you can do it again tomorrow because it is something you can and have done).

- Promotes optimism ('I can be healthier').

- It helps you to be kind to yourself – when you are having trouble with exercising, the first reaction is to get frustrated or angry with yourself, but if you have been 'listening' to this workbook, it is likely that you have started to coach, encourage and inspire yourself instead of beating yourself up.

- Helps you find pleasure in your body (it can do things you didn't realise).

- Helps you find pleasure in your environment (because you are out and about more).

Can you add any more benefits?

Over to You!

Being physically healthy does not need to involve overly vigorous workouts that are costly, intimidating or unsustainable. This chapter has emphasised the need to focus less on doing extreme workouts and more on reducing bouts of inactivity. We also explored how you can adopt a graded-exposure approach to physical activity by starting with something simple, such as walking, before progressing to moderate physical activities. Start simple, be realistic and stay in the company of people who are supportive of your goals.

Evaluate your perspective on physical well-being by reflecting on the following questions:

✎ **Have you had a previous experience of starting an exercise plan, but then stopped? Why do you think that happened and how could you prevent this happening again? For example, maybe you got lonely on your walks and could solve this problem with a walking buddy.**

_____

_____

_____

_____

_____

✎ **Are there factors or reasons that hold you back from doing any kind of physical activity? Consider potential solutions. For example, if you experience joint pain, maybe you could consider water aerobics, which is easier on the joints.**

_____

_____

_____

_____

_____

✎ What are your favourite ways of being physically active? How can you increase opportunities for these activities in your life? Perhaps you like dancing to music and could integrate this into your housework.

_____

_____

_____

_____

_____

✎ Remind yourself of Nudge Theory and the idea that you can change your environment to make physical activity the easier option. What nudges could you put in place to help you to be more active?

_____

_____

_____

_____

_____

Deciding on which exercises you can stick with has a lot to do with knowing your personal strengths and physical limitations. As with all areas of well-being discussed in this book, it is about working with your body, not against it.

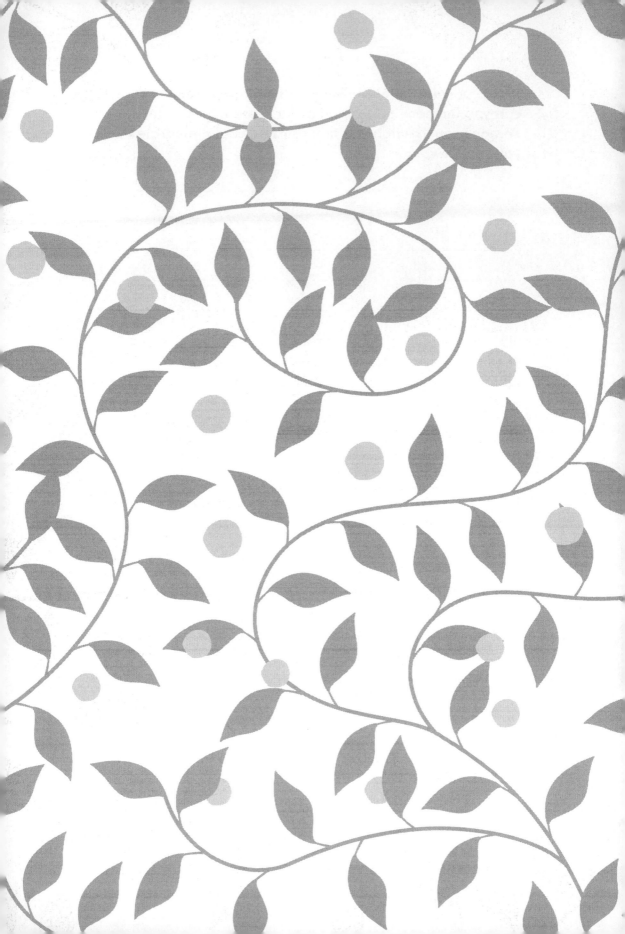

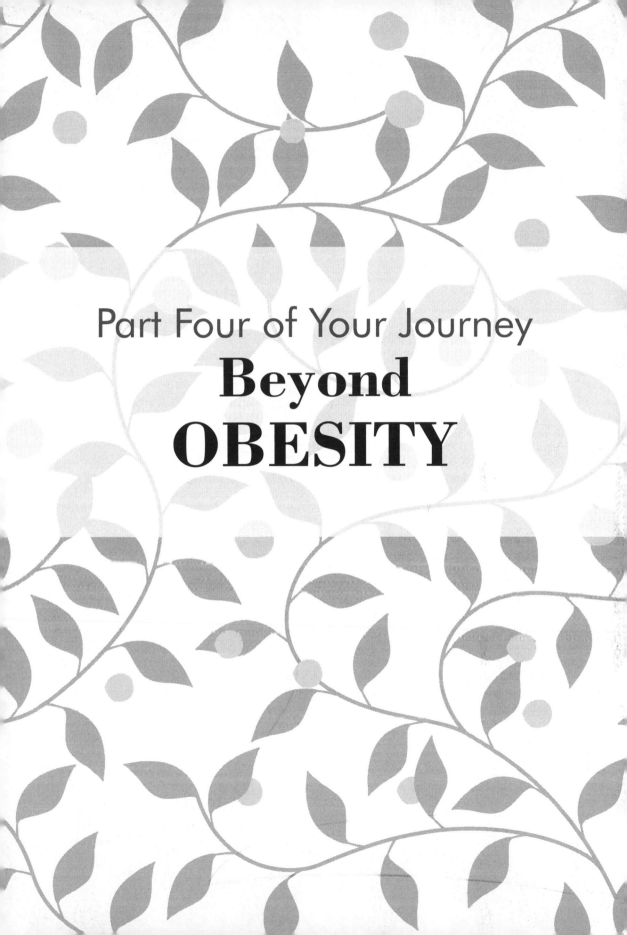

Part Four of Your Journey
Beyond
OBESITY

Chapter 14

Accepting Yourself

> *The curious paradox is that when I accept myself just as I am, then I can change.*
>
> Carl Rogers

There is often the expectation that once you lose weight you will feel better about yourself. However, many people who beat obesity are left with a negative self-image and low self-worth. Let's take a look at how you can learn to accept – and love – yourself.

Positive Body Image and Self-Worth

Body satisfaction is part of your overall body image, which can be very low in people with obesity and, often, in people who have beaten obesity. To achieve a positive body image and sense of self-worth, you need to first accept your body and, second, distance your self-worth from your weight – they aren't related.

Accepting your body (and appreciating it) can be hard after so many years of fighting it. However, practice makes perfect – even when it comes to accepting yourself. Here are some steps you can take to help gradually replace negative body image with a more positive one:

- Rather than compare yourself with others, appreciate other people for their differences.

- Don't rely on mirrors to judge yourself; just use them as practical aids for checking your hair or putting your make-up on.

- Look for beauty in personality and attitude, and decrease the focus on physical appearance.

- Avoid magazines that focus on appearance and body image, and choose ones that encourage physical and emotional well-being. If you feel bad about yourself after reading a magazine, it isn't the one for you.

- Only wear clothes that are comfortable and not too small or too big.

- Dress to express your personality and to bring out the real you.

- Don't weigh yourself, but use other markers to assess your progress with beating obesity or maintaining your weight loss, such as how you feel after physical activity and how your clothes feel.

- Spend time doing what makes you feel happy. You will be surprised how insignificant body size is as you become happier with your life.

- Respect your body. You might have experienced some difficulties with it, but just think of what it does for you – the places it gets you, the activities and pleasures it allows, and the potential it has.

Clothes were mentioned a couple of times in the list above because they have a powerful impact on self-esteem and body image. Make sure that you wear clothes that make you feel comfortable. Don't buy clothes that are too small and think of them as aspirational goals. This will only lead to negative feelings as you work towards fitting into them. Wear what makes you feel comfortable in the body you have now. Be kind to the body you have now. If you work with it, it will work with you. Yes, this might mean buying new clothes as your body changes and your self-esteem rises – but you deserve it. Would you have a loved one walking around in tight clothes that make them feel self-conscious or baggy clothes that make them feel untidy? Indeed, it goes both ways – as you and your body work together to beat obesity, you might find your clothes no longer feel comfortable because they are too big. Again, don't settle for anything other than clothes in which you feel content. Additionally, don't be afraid to create a signature style that exudes your growing confidence; this will enhance your feelings of self-worth further and emit an important message: 'I accept myself as I am – someone who is on a journey to become a healthier person.'

Self-Affirm Your Worth

What we tell ourselves – our affirmations – can shape who we are and how we see ourselves. If you tell yourself negative things, you will start to believe these negative stories. Fortunately, you can also use affirmations to turn negative beliefs, thoughts, ideas and self-talk into positive, empowering beliefs.

Affirmations can transform your life when practised regularly. They can help you turn from being your own worst enemy to your own best friend and self-healer.

The best affirmations:

- are about your personal qualities, not material 'things' (e.g. 'I am a caring person')

- are honest and directed inwards for you, not for what others want you to be (e.g. 'I feel I am considerate of other people's needs')

- are written or spoken with no negativity (e.g. 'I love myself')

- are repeated daily for at least 21 days in a row

- are about the present, even if the goal is for the future (e.g. 'Today, I feel good about myself').

Remember, what you feed your mind regularly through self-talk urges it to respond accordingly. Negative thoughts create unwanted realities, whereas positive self-talk creates empowering realities. Be just as vigilant with what you feed your mind as you have become with what you feed your body.

Practise affirmations daily and patiently; don't expect results straight away. It takes time to change a mindset. Here are some more tips:

- **Stay focused.** Be aware of any resistance you might experience, and be certain that your affirmations are genuine.

- **Welcome resistance.** There's nothing wrong with doubt. When flashes of self-doubt come, write them down and acknowledge them, but don't allow yourself to believe them.

- **Question.** When an affirmation still seems distant it might be worth questioning it. Ask: 'Whose affirmation is this really? Mine? My partner's, my father's or my manager's?' Your affirmations will only work if they come from you.

Behaviours or attitudes become habits if practised enough, just as we discussed in Chapter 10. The mind believes what it hears over and over. Therefore, it needs genuine, positive affirmations that bring out your personal qualities.

Be Thankful for What You Have

Another way to start accepting yourself is to look at those areas of your life that you are grateful for. Indeed, creating a gratitude list is a great way of achieving a realistic perception of yourself. Take the time to write down everything in your life that you are thankful for on a regular basis. When you are feeling particularly insecure, this is also a good exercise to remind yourself of the positive forces in your life. You can list all the talents you have, assets you possess and accomplishments in your life. Your gratitude list can also include the good things in your life such as the job you are enjoying, friends and family who care about you, or a beautiful house that you live in.

Don't Hold Off on Rewarding Yourself

Your weight is not an indicator of whether you are allowed to be kind to yourself or deserve to enjoy yourself. Don't put things you enjoy on hold until you reach your target goal. Allow yourself to enjoy the good things in life while you are on your journey. Life is for living; don't put off what you can do today – you deserve to enjoy life *now*. Recognising this will help you on your journey to a healthier lifestyle. The more enjoyment in your life, the happier you are likely to be. The happier you are, the more will and determination you will have to be kind to yourself and to maintain your new, healthier way of life.

Although it is motivating to structure your journey with rewards for various milestones, why not also include rewards that are independent of your progress towards beating obesity? Remember, beating obesity isn't just about weight; it is about learning to love yourself, respect yourself and be kind to yourself. It is a good idea to choose rewards that help build your self-esteem, such as having a spa day or buying a new outfit.

Rebrand Your Journey

I am hoping that by the time you have reached this chapter you will have started to see your journey to beat obesity not as a quest to lose weight but instead as a journey towards a healthier and happier self. Concentrate on the things that make your life more fulfilling rather than merely on what will help you lose weight or maintain your weight loss. By taking care of yourself, you will be showing respect for yourself, which naturally creates a desire to stay healthy. Ultimately, focus on *you*, not your weight. *You are much more than your weight.*

Track Your Progress

Tracking your progress is very important in your journey towards accepting yourself. Not only will this help you with positive reinforcement, it will also help you understand how you can become more effective at being the unique person that you are. Observing your small victories will be a great motivating factor and will propel you towards success – whatever that may look like for you. When you do observe your progress, take the time to praise yourself and reward yourself. This will help you associate progress with feelings of fulfilment and higher levels of self-esteem.

Don't Be Afraid of Overdoing It

Many people are taught to be modest and not be too self-involved. However, achieving a positive self-image will need you to be proactive about praising yourself. Although this can be extremely difficult for some people, especially those who have become accustomed to having a negative self-image, activities such as keeping a gratitude journal and listing good things about yourself can help turn things around. So don't be afraid of telling yourself out loud that you have great qualities. Speak up with confidence and make your quest public if the need arises. Many people put themselves down in public because they are taught that praising themselves is a vice. You need to let go of this feeling if you are already low on self-esteem, and work towards letting yourself and others know that you value yourself highly. If you treat yourself badly, you are giving others permission to do the same. The more you value yourself, the more others will value you.

Seek Professional Support

As you start to change on the outside due to your behavioural efforts, you might be surprised to find that certain aspects of your inner world have stayed the same. For example, if feelings of low self-worth and insecurities stem from your childhood rather than your weight, losing weight isn't going to solve all of your insecurities. If this is the case, you need to start by examining your past and understanding which specific events are having an impact on your self-worth. Once you understand them, you can work towards moving past them. Only when you let these negative feelings go can you start to fill that space with positive thoughts. If the past does play a dominating role in your sense of self-worth, consider counselling. Review Chapter 11 to assess whether this is something that might help. Even if you decided not to go down that route earlier, you might want to reconsider it now that you are ready to move forward with your life, especially if something is holding you back.

Over to You!

✎ To create affirmations that will work for you, list five areas of your life that you feel could be better.

1. _____

2. _____

3. _____

4. _____

5. _____

These might include your health, family life, friendships or self-esteem, examples of which include:

- Health – 'I listen to my body's need for nutritious foods.'

- Family – 'I am grateful for the lessons I have learned within my family.'

- Friendships – 'I choose to have my life filled with positive people.'

- Self-esteem – 'I believe in myself.'

Think about what needs to change to improve these aspects of your life – for example, asserting yourself with your family or developing confidence. Use these to help you come up with your affirmations:

- _____

- _____

- _____

- _____

- _____

Once you have written down your affirmations, aim to repeat them at least ten times each every day. As they start to make a positive difference in your life, you can replace them with other areas you want to work on.

✎ List five things that you are grateful for.

1. _____

2. _____

3. _____

4. _____

5. _____

✎ **Finally, list five things that you like about yourself.**

1. _____

2. _____

3. _____

4. _____

5. _____

As both your inner world and outer world start to change due to your hard work and dedication to creating a healthier life for yourself, you are likely to find yourself less focused on your issues with weight and more focused on what you want for your future. Let's explore this further in Chapter 15.

Chapter 15

The Future Is in Your Hands

> " *It is not in the stars to hold our destiny but in ourselves.*
>
> William Shakespeare "

Although it is important to focus on your journey to beat obesity, you need to remember that your life is about so much more. It is important not to let go of the other aspects of your life, especially as you enter the maintenance stage of your new healthy lifestyle. In fact, as you gain control over your weight and overall well-being, you are likely to feel propelled towards other aspects of life. With this in mind, let's take a look at your wider hopes and aspirations for life and start to shift your focus towards achieving these.

Rediscover Your Childhood Dreams

One very powerful exercise to help you create a clearer picture of your dreams is to take yourself back to when you were a child. This will allow your mind to focus by helping you to reconnect with those dreams and ideals you had when you were free of insecurities and other problems.

Ask yourself what you wanted to be when you grew up and what kind of a person you wanted to be. Although all those goals that you had as a child may not seem as appealing now, this exercise will help you compare your life now with a life when you were more carefree.

Once you have remembered your childhood dreams, pick out the ones that you still want to achieve. Include them in your journal and write out specific actions you can take to achieve these dreams. Review your notes regularly to keep track of your progress.

Here are some questions that can help you with this exercise:

- What are some of my earliest recollections of wanting to have a certain job or be in a certain role?

- What were my favourite activities as a child, and do I enjoy similar activities now?

- When was I happiest as a child, what was I doing and who was I with?

- Did I have any dreams or ambitions as I grew up?

- Which of these childhood dreams still appeal to me? What things can I do now that would be in the spirit of these childhood dreams?

- What would I say to the younger version of myself?

- What would the younger version of myself tell me about the dreams and hopes they have? Imagine a whole conversation between the two versions of yourself.

Answering these questions will help you clear your mind and recognise what is truly important to you. Although you may have changed over the years, the values that make up your character are likely to be similar.

What Are Your Hopes and Dreams for the Future?

Now that you have rediscovered the hopes and dreams you had as a child, let's take a closer look at your hopes and dreams now. Take some time to think about your hopes and dreams for the future. Don't hold back. Include anything, regardless of how feasible it seems at the moment.

- What do you want your life to be like?

- What would you like to be doing?

- Who will you be sharing your life with?

- What will your relationships look like?

- What kind of person are you in the future?

Visualising your answers to these questions can help you truly start to understand what you want from life, as visualisation brings emotions with it – warm feelings as you imagine your ideal world and ideal self. Whether you imagine two years from now, five years from now or ten years from now is up to you. There is no right or wrong way to explore your hopes and dreams for the future.

Next, consider how realistic these dreams are, before selecting the one you feel is most achievable. Take some time to consider what changes need to be made to help you reach that dream. For example, if a dream is to travel the world, maybe you need to save some money first! Repeat this exercise as you gain further confidence to grasp the many hopes and dreams you have identified.

Ultimately, your journey to an obesity-free life is only the beginning of your switch to a rewarding lifestyle. Although it's important to take care of your health, you need to make sure that you don't start ignoring other aspects of your life.

Finding Your Meaning

Meaning in life is about understanding your experiences and gaining a sense of purpose from them. It is unique to you because you create it. For many people who have struggled with obesity, their meaning in life has become to lose weight or be a certain desired weight. It has taken up so much time and energy that other priorities have been lost. However, here are some important reasons to find your meaning:

- People whose lives feel meaningful are driven by a sense of purpose. This helps them stick to their goals.

- Having meaning in life makes you see that you matter. It is vital for mental and physical well-being.

- People with meaningful lives are generally happier because they accept what life presents them with.

- Meaning in life protects you against the stresses and strains of daily living.

- When ordinary daily actions are surrounded by personal meaning, it lifts your sense of well-being.

Many people look for meaning in amazing events or they choose to wait for it to come to them rather than taking action to create meaning. Here are some ways you can add meaning to your life without having to wait:

- **Daily activities have meaning.** What you do on a daily basis – even small acts – can create meaning. For example, maybe your partner always gives you a kiss before leaving for work and this adds meaning to your life. Maybe you thoroughly enjoy your afternoon coffee with a good book, and this enhances your day.

- **Challenges have meaning.** Although you can't always prevent life's challenges, you can choose the way you think and react to such events. You can give difficult times a new, empowering meaning. For example, maybe you haven't found beating obesity easy, but what have the challenges given you? Maybe you appreciate certain activities more, or have greater passion for yourself.

Meaning is there to be made every day. All you need to do is look for it, and the best place to start is right where you are now as you embark on your journey beyond obesity!

Over to You!

✎ **Name five aspects of your life that you feel add meaning to your existence.**

1. _____
2. _____
3. _____
4. _____
5. _____

You might include something you are particularly good at or a person who you can't imagine life without. There are no right or wrong answers. This is *your* reality and *your* meaning.

✎ **Find a quiet place where you can sit down alone and focus on yourself. Make two lists. The first list is what you are good at. List everything that you can think of, even if it seems small – like making a great cup of tea.**

I am good at:

1. _____
2. _____
3. _____
4. _____
5. _____
6. _____
7. _____
8. _____
9. _____
10. _____

Aim for at least ten positives about yourself. At first you might find it difficult to come up with even five, but take your time and persist.

On the second list, write down what makes you happy, such as making someone smile or watching the sunrise.

I am happy when:

1. _____
2. _____
3. _____
4. _____
5. _____
6. _____
7. _____
8. _____
9. _____
10. _____

Both of these lists may need to be a work in progress and added to whenever you think of something new. At some point there is bound to be a link between something you are good at and something that makes you happy. Maybe there is someone who loves your cups of tea and it can make them smile during even the worst times. It's simple things like this that give our life meaning. Create your meaning and go for it!

This Is Your Beginning

> *Every ending is creating the space and opening for an amazing new beginning.*
>
> Bryan McGill

Congratulations on completing *I Can Beat Obesity!* If you have really engaged with this workbook and given it your all, you will have been on a journey. It might have even been a tough journey. But guess what? This isn't the end. It is only the beginning and you can choose where your new path will take you.

You might find you need to revisit various chapters of this workbook to keep you on track, and that is fine. This is what this workbook is there for – a companion to help you live the life you want and deserve – happy and healthy.

As we come to this juncture, I would like to wish you the very best as you embark on your new beginning – a new beginning which I hope will be enhanced by the tools you have gained from this workbook, especially the tool of self-care.

Good Luck and Good Health – You Can Beat Obesity!

Notes

Chapter 1

1. DeVille-Almond, J. (2015) 'NICE launches online learning tool on obesity.' Centre for Pharmacy Postgraduate Education Press Release. Available at www.cppe.ac.uk/news/a/489/nice-obesity-launched (accessed 5 July 2016).
2. World Health Organization (2016) 'Obesity and overweight.' Available at www.who.int/mediacentre/factsheets/fs311/en (accessed 5 July 2016).
3. World Health Organization 2016.
4. World Health Organization 2016.
5. Centers for Disease Control and Prevention (2015) 'Adult obesity facts.' Available at www.cdc.gov/obesity/data/adult.html (accessed 16 July 2016).
6. Public Health England (2016) 'About obesity.' National Obesity Observatory Publications. Available at www.noo.org.uk/NOO_about_obesity (accessed 16 July 2016).
7. National Health Service (2016) 'Obesity.' Available at www.nhs.uk/conditions/Obesity/Pages/Introduction.aspx (accessed 16 July 2016).
8. National Heart, Lung, and Blood Institute (2016) 'Classification of overweight and obesity by BMI, waist circumference, and associated disease risks.' Available at www.nhlbi.nih.gov/health/educational/lose_wt/BMI/bmi_dis.htm (accessed 16 July 2016).
9. World Health Organization 2016.
10. University of California Los Angeles (2016) 'Don't use body mass index to determine whether people are healthy, UCLA-led study says.' Available at http://newsroom.ucla.edu/releases/dont-use-body-mass-index-to-determine-whether-people-are-healthy-ucla-led-study-says (accessed 16 July 2016).
11. Ashwell, M. and Gibson, S. (2014) A proposal for a primary screening tool: 'Keep your waist circumference to less than half your height.' *BMC Medicine 12*, 207.
12. Diabetes.co.uk (2016) 'Visceral fat (active fat).' Available at www.diabetes.co.uk/body/visceral-fat.html (accessed 5 July 2016).
13. Diabetes.co.uk 2016.
14. Kershaw, E.E. and Flier, J.S. (2004) 'Adipose tissue as an endocrine organ.' *Journal of Clinical Endocrinology and Metabolism 89*, 6, 2548–2556.
15. Seale, P. and Lazar, M. (2009) 'Brown fat in humans: Turning up the heat on obesity.' *Diabetes 58*, 7, 1482–1484.
16. Doheny, K. (2009) 'The truth about fat.' WebMD Diet and Weight Management Feature Archive. Available at www.webmd.com/diet/the-truth-about-fat?page=1 (accessed 5 July 2016).

Chapter 2

1. Wardle, J. and Carnell, S. (2009) 'Appetite is a heritable phenotype associated with adiposity.' *Annual Behavioral Medicine 38*, 1, 25–30.
2. Fawcett, K. and Barroso, I. (2010) 'The genetics of obesity: FTO leads the way.' *Trends in Genetics 26*, 6, 266–274.
3. Abramson, E. (2006) *Body Intelligence*. New York: McGraw-Hill.
4. American Psychiatric Association (2013) 'Feeding and eating disorders.' Available at www.dsm5.org/documents/eating disorders fact sheet.pdf (accessed 16 July 2016).
5. Faith, M.S. and Kral, T.V.E. (2006) 'Social Environment and Genetic Influences in Obesity and Obesity-Promoting Behaviour: Fostering Research Integration.' In L.M. Hernandez and D.G. Blazer (eds) *Genes, Behavior, and the Social Environment: Moving Beyond the Nature/Nurture Debate*. Washington, DC: The National Academies Press.
6. Harmon, K. (2011) 'How obesity spreads in social networks.' *Scientific American* Online Health Article. Available at www.scientificamerican.com/article/social-spread-obesity (accessed 11 July 2016).
7. Nauert, R. (2012) 'Social networks influence obesity.' Psych Central News Article. Available at http://psychcentral.com/news/2012/07/10/social-networks-influence-obesity/41402.html (accessed 11 July 2016).
8. Christakis, N.A. and Fowler, J.H. (2007) 'The spread of obesity in a large social network over 32 years.' *New England Journal of Medicine 357*, 4, 370–379.
9. Christakis and Fowler 2007.
10. Nauert 2012.
11. Government Office for Science (2007) *Tackling Obesities: Future Choices – Obesogenic Environments – Evidence Review*. Available at www.gov.uk/government/uploads/system/uploads/attachment_data/file/295681/07-735-obesogenic-environments-review.pdf (accessed 11 July 2016).
12. Kahn, B.E. and Wansink, B. (2004) 'The influence of assortment structure on perceived variety and consumption quantities.' *Journal of Consumer Research 30*, 4, 519–533.

Chapter 3

1. Rand, C. and Macgregor, A. (1991) 'Successful weight loss following obesity surgery and the perceived liability of morbid obesity.' *International Journal of Obesity 15*, 9, 577–579.
2. Stanford Health Care (2015) 'Effects of obesity.' Available at https://stanfordhealthcare.org/medical-conditions/healthy-living/obesity.html (accessed 5 July 2016).
3. World Health Organization (2016) 'Cardiovascular diseases.' Available at www.who.int/topics/cardiovascular diseases/en (accessed 5 July 2016).
4. World Health Organization 2016.
5. American Diabetes Association (2015) 'Facts about type 2.' Available at www.diabetes.org/diabetes-basics/type-2/facts-about-type-2.html (accessed 5 July 2016).
6. American Diabetes Association 2015.
7. American Cancer Society (2016) 'Body weight and cancer risk.' Available at www.cancer.org/cancer/cancercauses/dietandphysicalactivity/bodyweightandcancerrisk/body-weight-and-cancer-risk-effects (accessed 5 July 2016).
8. American Cancer Society 2016.

9. National Health Service (2016) 'Obesity epidemic blamed for rise in womb cancer.' Available at www.nhs.uk/news/2016/04April/Pages/Obesity-epidemic-blamed-for-rise-in-womb-cancer-cases.aspx (accessed 5 July 2016).
10. Public Health England (2016) 'Maternal obesity.' Available at www.noo.org.uk/NOO_about_obesity/maternal_obesity_2015 (accessed 5 July 2016).
11. Public Health England 2016.
12. Obesity Society (2016) 'Obesity, bias, and stigmatization.' Available at www.obesity.org/obesity/resources/facts-about-obesity/bias-stigmatization (accessed 5 July 2016).
13. Obesity Society 2016.
14. Obesity Society 2016.
15. Markowitz, S., Friedman, M.A. and Arent, S.M. (2008) 'Understanding the relation between obesity and depression: Causal mechanisms and implications for treatment.' *Clinical Psychology: Science and Practice 15*, 1, 1–20.
16. Luppino, F.S., de Wit, L.M., Bouvy, P.F., Stijnen, T. *et al.* (2010) 'Overweight, obesity, and depression: A systematic review and meta-analysis of longitudinal studies.' *Archives of General Psychiatry 67*, 3, 220–229.
17. Pratt, L.A. and Brody, D.J. (2014) 'Depression and obesity in the U.S. adult household population, 2005–2010.' National Center for Health Statistics Data Brief No. 167. Available at www.cdc.gov/nchs/products/databriefs/db167.htm (accessed 5 July 2016).
18. Luppino *et al.* 2010.
19. Baumeister, H. and Harter, M. (2007) 'Mental disorders in patients with obesity in comparison with healthy probands.' *International Journal of Obesity 31*, 7, 1155–1164; Scott, K., Bruffaerts, R., Simon, G.E., Alonso, J. *et al.* (2008) 'Obesity and mental disorders in the general population: Results from the world mental health surveys.' *International Journal of Obesity 32*, 1, 192–200.
20. Mayo Clinic (2015) 'Anxiety.' Available at www.mayoclinic.org/diseases-conditions/anxiety/home/ovc-20168121 (accessed 5 July 2016).
21. Forhan, F. and Gill, S. (2013) 'Obesity, functional mobility and quality of life.' *Best Practice and Research Clinical Endocrinology and Metabolism 27*, 2, 129–137.

Chapter 4

1. Johns, D.J., Hartmann-Boyce, J., Jebb, S.A. and Aveyard, P. (2014) 'Diet or exercise interventions vs combined behavioral weight management programs: A systematic review and meta-analysis of direct comparisons.' *Journal of the Academy of Nutrition and Dietetics 114*, 10, 1557–1568.
2. Zelman, K. (2007) '8 Ways To Think Thin.' WebMD Diet and Weight Management Feature Archive. Available at www.webmd.com/diet/obesity/8-ways-to-think-thin (accessed 5 July 2016).
3. Agency for Healthcare Research and Quality (2014) 'Community Connections: Linking primary care patients to local resources for better management of obesity.' Available at www.ahrq.gov/professionals/prevention-chronic-care/improve/community/obesity-toolkit/obtoolkit-tool14.html (accessed 11 July 2016).

Chapter 5

1. DiClemente, C.C. and Prochaska, J.O. (1988) 'Toward a Comprehensive Transtheoretical Model of Change: Stages of Change and Addictive Behaviors.' In W.R. Miller and N. Heather (eds) *Treating Addictive Behaviors, Second Edition*. New York: Plenum Press; Prochaska, J.O., Norcross, J.C. and DiClemente, C.C. (2007) *Changing for Good*. New York: Harper Collins.
2. Prochaska, J.O. and DiClemente, C.C. (1992) 'Stages of Change in the Modification of Problem Behaviors.' In M. Hersen, R.M. Eisler and P.M. Miller (eds) *Progress in Behavior Modification*. Sycamore, IL: Sycamore Press.
3. Prochaska and DiClemente 1992.
4. Smart Recovery (2016) 'Understanding the stages of change.' Self-Management and Recovery Training Resources (from Prochaska, Norcross and DiClemente, *Changing for Good*). Available at www.smartrecovery.org/resources/library/Articles_and_ Essays/Stages_of_Change/understanding_stages_of_change.htm (accessed 16 July 2016).

Chapter 6

1. Bandura, A. (1994). 'Self-efficacy.' In V.S. Ramachaudran (ed.) *Encyclopedia of Human Behavior, Volume 4*. New York: Academic Press.
2. University of Michigan Medical School (2016) 'Weight Efficacy Lifestyle questionnaire.' Available at www.med.umich.edu/intmed/endocrinology/ weightmanagement/ShortForm-WeightEfficacyLifestyleQuestionnaire.pdf (accessed 16 July 2016).
3. Digate Muth, N. (2015) 'Coaching behavior change toolbox: The confidence ruler.' American Council on Exercise Professional Resources. Available at www.acefitness. org/prosourcearticle/5627/coaching-behavior-change-toolbox-the (accessed 16 July 2016).
4. Digate Muth 2015.
5. Warziski, M.T., Sereika, S.M., Styn, M.A., Music, E. and Burke, L.E. (2008) 'Changes in self-efficacy and dietary adherence. The impact on weight loss in the PREFER study.' *Journal of Behavioral Medicine 31*, 1, 81–92; Shin, H., Shin, J., Liu, P.Y., Dutton, G.R., Abood, D.A. and Ilich, J.Z. (2011) 'Self-efficacy improves weight loss in overweight/obese postmenopausal women during a 6-month weight loss intervention.' *Nutrition Research 31*, 11, 822–828.
6. Warziski et al. 2008.
7. Shin et al. 2011.
8. Bandura, A. (1997) *Self-Efficacy: The Exercise of Control*. New York: W.H. Freeman.
9. Bandura 1997.
10. Bandura 1997.

Chapter 7

1. Cullen, K.W., Baranowski, T. and Smith, S.P. (2001) 'Using goal setting as a strategy for dietary behaviour change.' *Journal of the American Dietetic Association 101*, 5, 562–566.

2. Strecher, V.J., Seijts, G.H., Kok, G.J., Latham, G.P. *et al.* (1995) 'Goal setting as a strategy for health behavior change.' *Health Education Quarterly 22*, 2, 190–200.
3. Shilts, M.K., Horowitz, M. and Townsend, M.S. (2004) 'Goal setting as a strategy for dietary and physical activity behavior change: A review of the literature.' *American Journal of Health Promotion 19*, 2, 81–93.
4. Haughey, D. (2016) 'Smart goals.' Project Smart: Project Management Resources. Available at www.projectsmart.co.uk/smart-goals.php (accessed 8 July 2016).
5. Haughey, D. (2014) 'A brief history of SMART goals.' Project Smart: Project Management Resources. Available at www.projectsmart.co.uk/brief-history-of-smart-goals.php (accessed 8 July 2016).
6. Wood, W. (2014) 'How we form habits, change existing ones.' Society for Personality and Social Psychology Article, Science Daily. Available at www.sciencedaily.com/releases/2014/08/140808111931.htm (accessed 8 July 2016).

Chapter 8

1. Singh, M. (2014) 'Mood, food, and obesity.' *Frontiers in Psychology 5*, 925, 1–20.
2. Hanly, L. (2015) 'Foods that trigger the release of dopamine.' Livestrong Food and Health Articles. Available at www.livestrong.com/article/64566-foods-trigger-release-dopamine (accessed 6 July 2016).
3. American Psychological Association (2013) 'Stress and eating.' Available at www.apa.org/news/press/releases/stress/2013/eating.aspx (accessed 6 July 2016).
4. American Psychological Association 2013.
5. Mayo Clinic (2015) 'Weight loss: Gain control of emotional eating.' Available at www.mayoclinic.org/healthy-lifestyle/weight-loss/in-depth/weight-loss/art-20047342 (accessed 6 July 2016).
6. MedHelp (2016) 'Track your mood.' Available at www.medhelp.org/land/mood-tracker (accessed 11 July 2016).
7. MoodPanda (2016) MoodPanda Happiness Tracking website and app for iPhone and Android. Available at www.moodpanda.com (accessed 11 July 2016).
8. Vivyan, C. (2010) 'Mood Diary 2.' Self-help and therapist resources. Available at http://get.gg/docs/MoodDiary2.pdf (accessed 11 July 2016).
9. Vivyan, C. (2015) 'Mood Diary.' Available at www.getselfhelp.co.uk/docs/MoodDiary.pdf (accessed 16 July 2016).
10. Purcell, M. (2015) 'The health benefits of journaling.' Psych Central Library. Available at http://psychcentral.com/lib/the-health-benefits-of-journaling (accessed 8 July 2016).
11. Kaiser Permanente (2008) 'Keeping a food diary doubles diet weight loss, study suggests.' Science Daily. Available at www.sciencedaily.com/releases/2008/07/080708080738.htm (accessed 6 July 2016).
12. Manzoni, G., Pagnini, F., Gorini, A., Preziosa, A. *et al.* (2009) 'Can relaxation training reduce emotional eating in women with obesity? An exploratory study with 3 months of follow-up.' *Journal of the American Dietetic Association 109*, 8, 1427–1432.
13. Singh, N.N., Lancioni, G.E., Singh, A.N., Winton, A.S.W. *et al.* (2008) 'A mindfulness-based health wellness program for managing morbid obesity.' *Clinical Case Studies 7*, 4, 327–339.
14. O'Reilly, G.A., Cook, L., Spruijt-Metz, D. and Black, D.S. (2014) 'Mindfulness-based interventions for obesity-related eating behaviours: A literature review.' *Obesity Reviews 15*, 6, 453–461.
15. Singh *et al.* 2008.

Chapter 9

1. Fuhr, L. (2015) '4 mental roadblocks that sabotage weight loss.' Popsugar Health and Fitness Blog. Available at www.popsugar.com.au/fitness/Mental-Thoughts-Sabotage-Weight-Loss-33610673 (accessed 6 July 2016).
2. Cognitive Behavioral Therapy Los Angeles (2015) 'Common cognitive distortions: Mind reading.' Available at http://cogbtherapy.com/cbt-blog/common-cognitive-distortions-mind-reading (accessed 6 July 2016).
3. European Food Information Council (2015) 'Black and white thinking may hinder one's ability to maintain a healthy weight.' Available at www.eufic.org/page/en/show/latest-science-news/fftid/black_and_white_thinking_may_hinder_one_s_ability_to_maintain_a_healthy_weight (accessed 6 July 2016).
4. European Food Information Council 2015.
5. Hamid, T. (2009) *Thinking in Circles about Obesity: Applying Systems Thinking to Weight Management*. eBook: Springer Science + Business Media.
6. Grohol, J.M. (2015) 'What is catastrophizing?' Psych Central Library. Available at http://psychcentral.com/lib/what-is-catastrophizing (accessed 6 July 2016).
7. Flintoff, J. (2014) 'How to silence negative thinking.' *The Guardian* Online. Available at www.theguardian.com/lifeandstyle/2014/aug/11/how-to-silence-negative-thinking (accessed 6 July 2016).
8. Covey, S.R. (2016) 'The 7 habits of highly effective people. Habit 2: Begin with the end in mind.' Available at www.stephencovey.com/7habits/7habits-habit2.php (accessed 6 July 2016).
9. Mendell, J. (2015) 'These 6 common thoughts are making you gain weight.' *Women's Health Magazine* Online Blog. Available at www.womenshealthmag.com/weight-loss/can-negative-thoughts-cause-weight-gain (accessed 6 July 2016).

Chapter 10

1. Wood, W. (2014) 'How we form habits, change existing ones.' Society for Personality and Social Psychology article, Science Daily. Available at www.sciencedaily.com/releases/2014/08/140808111931.htm (accessed 8 July 2016).
2. London School of Economics (2014) 'Nudging the obese.' Available at www.lse.ac.uk/researchAndExpertise/researchHighlights/Health/NudgingTheObese.aspx (accessed 10 July 2016).

Chapter 11

1. Avena, N. and Talbott, J. (2014) *Why Diets Fail (Because You're Addicted to Sugar)*. New York: Ten Speed Press.
2. Lecaros-Bravo, J., Cruzat-Mandich, C., Diaz-Castrillon, F. and Moore-Infante, C. (2015) 'Bariatric surgery in adults: Variables that facilitate and hinder weight loss from patients' perspective.' *Nutricion Hospitalaria 31*, 4, 1504–1512.
3. Chibucos, T.R., Leite, R.W. and Weis, D.L. (2005) *Readings in Family Theory*. Thousand Oaks, CA: Sage Publications.

Chapter 12

1. Aamodt, S. (2016) *Why Diets Make Us Fat*. New York: Penguin Random House.
2. Gunnars, K. (2016) 'Food addiction – a serious problem with a simple solution.' Authority Nutrition. Available at https://authoritynutrition.com/how-to-overcome-food-addiction (accessed 6 July 2016).
3. McCready Hart, L. (2011) 'Dr. David Kessler, author of *The End of Overeating*, on why we can't stop eating.' *Huffington Post* Wellness Blog. Available at www.huffingtonpost.com/entry/d-kessler-author-of-emthe_b_195676 (accessed 16 July 2016).
4. Mole, B. (2016) 'Gut microbes send message to the brain that sparks obesity in rodents.' ARS Technica. Available at http://arstechnica.com/science/2016/06/in-rodents-fed-high-fat-diets-gut-microbes-boost-hunger-trigger-obesity (accessed 6 July 2016).
5. Sarlio-Lähteenkorva, S. (2015) 'Could a sugar tax help combat obesity?' *BMJ 2015*, 351, h4047.
6. Oates, A.E. (2014) 'The weight issue: It is not due to a lack of willpower.' British Obesity Society Blog. Available at http://britishobesitysociety.tumblr.com/post/92454315939/the-weight-issue-it-is-not-due-to-a-lack-of (accessed 6 July 2016).
7. Public Health England (2016) 'New Eatwell Guide illustrates a healthy, balanced diet.' Press Release. Available at www.gov.uk/government/news/new-eatwell-guide-illustrates-a-healthy-balanced-diet (accessed 6 July 2016).
8. Public Health England 2016.
9. Harvard School of Public Health (2016) 'Healthy weight checklist.' Obesity Prevention Source. Available at www.hsph.harvard.edu/obesity-prevention-source/diet-lifestyle-to-prevent-obesity (accessed 12 July 2016).
10. Bates College Health Center (2012) 'Mindful eating diary.' Available at www.bates.edu/health/files/2012/04/Mindful-Eating-Diary.pdf (accessed 6 July 2016).
11. Nourish Move Thrive California (2014) 'Harness your inner wisdom with a hunger scale.' Available at http://nourishmovethrive.ca/articles/harness-your-inner-wisdom-hunger-scale (accessed 12 July 2016).
12. Grover, J. (2013) 'Mindful eating: 5 easy tips to get started.' Mother Nature Network. Available at www.mnn.com/food/healthy-eating/stories/mindful-eating-5-easy-tips-to-get-started (accessed 6 July 2016).
13. Aamodt 2016.
14. Ross, C. (2013) 'So you think you're eating mindfully.' Psychology Today. Available at www.psychologytoday.com/blog/real-healing/201309/so-you-think-youre-eating-mindfully (accessed 12 July 2016).
15. Obesity Action Coalition (2016) *What is Mindful Eating?* Available at www.obesityaction.org/wp-content/uploads/04_Mindful_Eating.pdf (accessed 30 August 2016).
16. Intelligent Eating (2014) 'Intelligent Eating – If you have your health, you have everything.' Available at www.intelligenteating.org (accessed 6 July 2016).

Chapter 13

1. Health and Social Care Information Centre (2015) *Statistics on Obesity, Physical Activity and Diet*. Leeds: Health and Social Care Information Centre. Available at www.hscic.gov.uk/catalogue/PUB16988/obes-phys-acti-diet-eng-2015.pdf (accessed 12 July 2016).
2. Department of Health (2011) *Physical Activity Guidelines for Adults (19–64 Years)*, Fact Sheet 4. Available at www.gov.uk/government/uploads/system/uploads/attachment_data/file/213740/dh_128145.pdf (accessed 12 July 2016).
3. Health and Social Care Information Centre 2015.
4. Wayne State University Physician Group (2011) 'The role of exercise in treating obesity.' Available at www.wsupgdocs.org/family-medicine/WayneStateContentPage.aspx?nd=1571 (accessed 12 July 2016).
5. Morris, K. (2015) 'Exercising dangers for obese people.' Livestrong Sports and Fitness Articles. Available at www.livestrong.com/article/554136-exercising-dangers-for-obese-people (accessed 12 July 2016).
6. Morrison, S. (2014) 'Take small steps to get active and lose weight.' British Obesity Society Weight Loss Post. Available at http://britishobesitysociety.tumblr.com/post/88360837889/take-small-steps-to-get-active-and-lose-weight (accessed 12 July 2016).
7. Morrison 2014.
8. Stewart, G. (2014) 'How to make walking really work for you.' British Obesity Society Weight Loss Post. Available at http://britishobesitysociety.tumblr.com/post/89655296037/how-to-make-walking-really-work-for-you (accessed 12 July 2016).
9. Kellow, J. (2016) 'Dieting and metabolism.' Weight Loss Resources UK. Available at www.weightlossresources.co.uk/calories/burning_calories/starvation.htm (accessed 16 July 2016).
10. American Osteopathic Association (2016) 'Battling boredom in your workout.' Available at www.osteopathic.org/osteopathic-health/about-your-health/health-conditions-library/general-health/Pages/workout-boredom.aspx (accessed 16 July 2016).

Dr Nicola Davies is a health psychologist, counsellor, and medical writer specialising in raising awareness about health and well-being. She is a member of the British Psychological Society and the British Association for Counselling and Psychotherapy. Nicola also keeps a health psychology blog and runs an online forum for counsellors. Nicola is the co-author of the *Eating Disorder Recovery Handbook*, also published by Jessica Kingsley Publishers.